Hospitals, Health, and People

Hospitals, Health, and People

Albert W. Snoke, M.D.

Yale University Press
New Haven and London

Designed by James J. Johnson
and set in Palatino types by
The Publishing Nexus Incorporated, Guilford, Connecticut
Printed in the United States of America by
Murray Printing Company, Westford, Massachusetts.

Library of Congress Cataloging-in-Publication Data

Snoke, Albert W. (Albert Waldo), 1907–
    Hospitals, health, and people.

    Includes index.
    1. Hospitals—Administration. 2. Snoke, Albert W.
(Albert Waldo), 1907—   . 3. Hospital administrators—
United States—Biography. I. Title. [DNLM: 1. Delivery
of Health Care. 2. Health Facility Administrators.
3. Health Planning. 4. Hospital Administration.
WX 150 S673h]
RA971.S657   1987   362.1'1'068   86–24631
ISBN 0–300–03588–8 (alk. paper)

The paper in this book meets the guidelines for permanence
and durability of the Committee on Production Guidelines
for Book Longevity of the Council on Library Resources.

10 9 8 7 6 5 4 3 2 1

I dedicate this book to Parnie Hamilton Storey Snoke, M.D., M.P.H.
"Al-and-Parnie" was a single word in the lexicon of
the hospital community for over forty years. Parnie was the partner and
colleague, wife and friend, with whom I traveled the long road
described in this book, always together until her death in 1981.
The events set forth here would never have happened without her.
She brought me to an understanding of the true dimensions
of health care for people.
I can only add the toast that Parnie and I
drank every evening in our later years:

"To those we love, wherever they may be."

Contents

Acknowledgments

Several individuals and organizations provided invaluable assistance in the production of this book.

First and foremost is Edward Tripp of the Yale University Press. He first suggested that I write about hospital administration, suffered through my initial efforts, and edited the first seven chapters.

James Hague, retired editor of the journal *Hospitals*, also edited, reviewed, revised, and cut the manuscript down to size.

Alexander McMahon, retired president of the American Hospital Association, provided AHA funds for secretarial support. Eloise Foster, head librarian at the AHA Bacon Library, and her staff did valuable research and provided much of my supporting data.

Eilleen Reilly typed the many drafts of the manuscript and checked it for accuracy.

Stef Jones at Yale University Press edited—and sometimes rewrote—the final draft.

I would also like to thank Dr. Mitchell Rabkin, the reader for Yale University Press.

Introduction

Several years ago, Edward Tripp, then editor-in-chief of the Yale University Press, suggested that I write a book on hospital administration. I declined for a number of reasons, the principal one being that hospital administration is a constantly changing discipline. However, as I thought of the suggestion during the following year, I began to realize that I had participated in a revolutionary period in health care in this country. I also saw that my experience epitomized the transition from a physician's firm dedication to diagnosing and treating a patient's *disease* to a broader concern for the patient himself, as a fellow human being who is part of a family and a community and who is affected by the many stresses that face people in our society today.

This experience was a gradual educational process. Though I didn't know it at the time, I was fortunate to start my career with one of the giants in hospital administration, Dr. Basil MacLean. Through his support and influence I came to know many of his predecessors as well as his contemporaries, all leaders in the health services. As a physician, associated with prestigious medical centers in Rochester and later in New Haven, I was able to participate in many decisions on major health and welfare issues of state and national significance. In writing of these issues, I am afraid that I have occasionally found it hard to separate my personal involvement in some of the resulting confrontations from the broader social issues.

In recalling years of changing responsibilities and relationships, I find that I have produced a chronicle of my "post-graduate" education in the care of people—an account that seems to fall naturally into the distinct phases to which I have referred in the text. I believe, however, that the final stage of my evolving view of people care can best be typified by the picture of the small statuette *Discharged Cured* that Dr. Jack Masur gave me in the late 1940s. I hung it on the wall of my office at the Yale-New Haven Hospital and again in my office when I was an adviser to the governor of Illinois. It is now in my study at home. Each year I took this picture to my seminar in the course on hospital administration at Yale and spent the entire period discussing what the picture implies about our responsibilities in caring for people. I was most flattered recently to see a copy of this picture on the office wall of one of my former students, who now heads a major university teaching hospital.

I can do no better in explaining what this picture means to me than to quote from an article by Dr. Masur, "Some Challenges in Hospital Administration," that appeared in the *Journal of Medical Education* 30, no. 10 (October 1955), pages 567–72.

The whole question of the responsibility of the physician, of the hospital, of the health agency, brings vividly to my mind a small statue which I saw a great many years ago on the mantle in the late Dr. Corwin's office at the New York Academy of Medicine—a statue of a patient discharged from a hospital:

It is a pathetic little figure of a man, coat collar turned up and shoulders hunched against the chill winds, clutching his belongings in a paper bag—shaking, tremulous, discouraged. He's clearly unfit for work—no employer would dare to take a chance on hiring him. You know that he will need much more help before he can face the world with shoulders back and confidence in himself. You suspect that he may never be able to go back to the work he has done before his illness. Past the age of 50, he will have to learn how to do a different kind of work if he is to be self-supporting. You think that he was probably once the responsible breadwinner of a family, husband and father, proud of his ability to earn enough to feed, clothe and educate his children. Now his present weakness is shaking him; his self-respect is deeply damaged. He is discouraged and frightened. This is the man who has been discharged with the cryptic notation on his medical chart: Discharged—Cured.

The statuette epitomizes the task of medical rehabilitation: to bridge the gap between the sick and a job. Those of us who work in hospitals must join with education, social work, employment placement, vocational guidance and any number of related services to provide patients with the help they need to restore them to their maximum functioning. It means that, more than ever, physicians in hospitals must realize that their job is not ended when the fever is down, or the sutures out or "clinical cure" has been achieved. It means that rehabilitation does not limit itself to amputees or paraplegics, but that we need to think in terms of the bookkeeper with glaucoma, the welder with diabetes, the furrier with asthma and the truck driver with diminishing hearing. It means that we shall have to concentrate on the ends as well as the means in the management of patients.

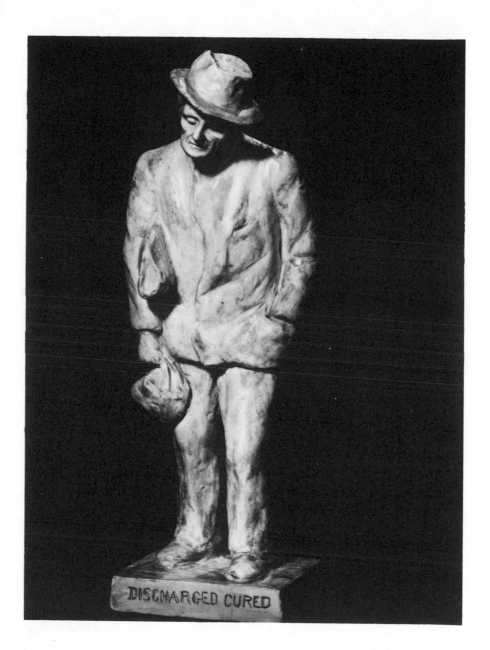

DISCHARGED CURED

1

The Hospital Administrator

In the early 1930s, as a medical student and a member of the resident staff at the Stanford-Lane University Hospital in San Francisco, I took a dim view of its administrator. He was remote, he never seemed to smile, and, when one had an occasion to talk to him, he usually said, "No!" All he seemed to think about was saving money and deferring to the medical staff. In 1936–37, when I was the resident in pediatrics at Strong Memorial Hospital (SMH) in Rochester, New York, the house staff still discussed with derision a former assistant administrator who spent his spare time flushing toilets in the interns' quarters and measuring with a stopwatch the time the water ran, to ensure economy.

Forty-five years later, the hospital administrator still seems remote and his or her responsibilities are still ill defined. Attempts to clarify them have resembled those of the fabled blind men who argued over the definition of an elephant after each had touched just one part of the animal. To many he or she appears to be concerned only with operating and balancing the budget of an institution that provides "sickness care," instead of having a basic concern for people's health. The hospital administrator is depicted on television and on film as a harried superintendent, busy with dollars, public relations, and marketing, and unduly deferential to senior physicians and influential members of the community.

My experiences in Rochester and in New Haven helped me to identify the many responsibilities that a hospital administrator was expected to assume, to establish their priorities, and to decide who should be responsible for carrying them out. The responsibilities of the administrator concerned with operating the institution and keeping it viable were obviously important. These included long-range planning (its title now upgraded to "strategic planning"), recruiting and retaining experienced personnel, maintaining good relations with medical staff and board, coping with governmental regulations, implementing community programs, creating reimbursement formulas, and capital financing. Finally, I was introduced to the issues that preoccupy those concerned with health today—cost containment, program management, competition, marketing, and corporate reorganization.

Although I was personally involved with all of these issues, I learned that part of my management responsibility was to delegate many of them to associates who had greater expertise in those areas. This allowed me time to be concerned with the care of the patient both in the hospital and in the community. I came to believe this responsibility can best be assumed by the chief executive officer (CEO) of the hospital because he or she is in the best position to see the overall picture. Moreover, no one else has as much authority to correct inadequacies and implement constructive programs coordinating the many diverse departments in a hospital.

Thus I suspect that my interest in making the hospital an instrument for promoting *health* and in creating a friendly and helpful atmosphere were the primary reasons for my remaining in hospital administration after I had accepted Basil MacLean's offer to make me assistant director of Strong Memorial Hospital in Rochester, New York. I agreed originally to try it for two years. But I quickly came to feel that my position in the administration of a major hospital would enable me to make a farther-ranging contribution to "people care" than I could as an individual practitioner of medicine. But it took some time for me to rationalize this attitude even to myself—to say nothing of my former classmates who accused me of prostituting four years of medical school and five years of residency training to become a damned hospital administrator.

My convictions were developed gradually in the administrative environment in which I first worked, at Strong Memorial Hospital in Rochester. Dr. MacLean met every weekday morning with his administrative staff, the director of nursing, and the head of the admitting office. There we discussed the events of the previous day and explored problems in the operation of the hospital, particularly those related to patient care. After the admitting officer and the chief nurse had left, administrative activities were reviewed. Dr. MacLean was deeply involved in local and national hospital and Blue Cross affairs, and his perspective provided a true learning experience for his staff.

When I moved to New Haven in 1946, I took Dr. MacLean's ideas and practices with me. I was interested in how patients were being cared for, in the operation of the hospital as it pertained to these patients, and in the difficulties that arose when department heads and assistants wanted to bring about improvements. I wanted, with their help, to run a better hospital—one that was concerned with people care. My experiences in Rochester and the even more complicated problems I encountered in a university teaching hospital that was not owned by the university, and that also served as a community and a municipal hospital, continued to impress upon me the unique impact the director could have upon health care. A hospital was typically thought of as a place one came to die—a "house of failure," as one of my British colleagues described our hospital, to my great indignation. The challenge to make such an institution a place not just to treat sickness, but also to promote health, persuaded me to remain in hospital administration. Because a hospital stay is only a short, acute (and expensive) episode in the continuum of health and illness, I hoped to extend the hospital's function and influence to providing health care for those outside it. More than a hospital administrator, I wanted to be a *health administrator*, and as such to make an even greater contribution to the well-being of people in the hospital as well as in the community.

In fairness, however, as I look back upon my approximately fifty years' association with hospitals, I must say that I understand hospital administrators' preoccupation with the fiscal, administrative, and organizational aspects of their jobs. The hospital cannot exist for long if it is not solvent, or if it cannot meet the needs of its patients or its staff. Therefore, I comment on the operational aspects of hospitals before discussing further the primary responsibility of the hospital or health administrator—the care of the people.

INN-KEEPING

At the 1939 American Hospital Association (AHA) convention, Basil MacLean suggested that the god Janus be considered the patron saint of the hospital administrators, because he was two-faced and probably related to janitors. Although indignation was loudly voiced, there was, and remains, some truth in the comment. Dr. MacLean was not entirely fair, however, in heaping such scorn upon hospital administrators, who seem so preoccupied with hotel-keeping and with money.

The hospital administrator must see that the many traditional "hotel functions" of the hospital are carried out—patients must be housed while being cared for. These aspects of hospital management are highly visible and readily subject to public criticism. Room furnishings, cleanliness, food, reception, the business office, the atmosphere, and the final bill are subjects that laypeople think they can understand and judge. The patient is rare, however, who has any concept of the functions or cost of operating rooms, laboratories, or medical, nursing, and special services.

I still react with indignation to the oft-repeated phrase, "I can get better service in a room at the Waldorf-Astoria at much less cost." In 1951, this attitude led me and my associates to publish a booklet that compared costs of hotel and hospital services. Housekeeping, maintenance, laundry, heat and electricity, telephone service, information services, insurance, and so on accounted for only 31 percent of per diem hospital costs, but they made up all of the costs of a hotel room. The costs of nursing, food, and a broad array of special services made up 69 percent of hospital charges. These services are, of course, the real reason for the hospital's existence. The late John Knowles, general director of the Massachusetts General Hospital (MGH) from 1962 to 1971, also became tired of the continuing hotel/hospital comparisons. He calculated that the "hotel" costs at MGH in the mid-1960s accounted for 11.3 percent of the total bill—even smaller than the proportion I had calculated in 1951.

FISCAL RESPONSIBILITY

Realistic fiscal and personnel management and the kind of administrative organization required for satisfactory operation have been a long time coming to hospitals. Even in the 1940s, many hospitals functioned under the aegis of Lord and Lady Bountiful or by rattling the tin cup to cover the deficits, and hospital administrators were almost always required to be penny-pinchers. Prior to the pioneering work done by the Cleveland Hospital Council in 1932, there was no standard chart of accounts for hospitals. Yearly budgets either did not exist or were produced in an afternoon. In 1935, C. Rufus Rorem and Basil MacLean drafted what eventually became the approved Manual of Hospital Accounting and Statistics for the AHA.

My education in fiscal responsibility started when I came to New Haven in 1946, and for years I felt that I was a laggard in this area. To my amazement, I have learned that some of my most respected colleagues have only recently developed realistic budgets for their hospitals and medical schools. Apparently, they felt that administration was easier without fixed budgets—or, as one dean confided to me twenty years ago, "It is much easier to work with my associates if I can keep things a little fuzzy."

Personnel Management

Personnel administration and corporate management are two other issues that have grown in importance during the past forty years and now are presenting formidable competition to the hospital administrator's basic responsibility for care of the patient. In the late 1930s, personnel administration was in an embryonic phase. At the first meeting of the Medical Administrators Conference in 1939, nine young physicians—all assistant administrators in major hospitals in the East—spent a great deal of time on the subject of the "Personnel Director: What is his place and program in your organization?" All were just beginning to consider creating such a post in their hospitals.

In the past, the hospital was a philanthropic institution. For years hospitals could take care of poor people because their costs were low, physicians provided their services without charge, and many could rely on fund drives, Community Chest funds, or individual donors to make up deficits. Unfortunately, the employees, as well as the overcharged private patients, were involuntary philanthropists. Student nurses were exploited, employees were paid extremely low wages, and such things as pensions were not even considered.

When I came to New Haven, I was profoundly impressed by the large number of elderly men and women who were working in the housekeeping and dietary departments. Many were in their middle or late seventies and were not particularly effective. I wondered why the hospital was not retiring them and and hiring younger people. The answer was simple: there was no pension system, only a custom that, when a person retired, he or she was paid twenty dollars a month. The administration knew that these people couldn't live on such a "pension," so they were kept on beyond their retirement age so that they could make enough money to live on. A pension plan was soon instituted, but it was not easy. Not only did many employees need to have their back benefits financed, but the increased cost also had to be reimbursed. Niggardly reimbursement rates and the availability of people to work at low wages, as well as lack of interest and expertise in personnel management, meant that years passed before any attention was paid to productivity or retirement benefits.

I was slow to recognize the responsibility of the hospital administrator or the CEO to address the very important issue of minority rights. Raised in a small town in Washington and educated to become a physician, I was innocent of problems related to color, race, or creed until after I became involved in hospital administration. Even then, at Rochester and New Haven, only isolated instances, such as the admission of the first black woman to the SMH School of Nursing had much impact upon my social consciousness.

The passage of the Civil Rights Act in 1964 brought the matter into sharper focus as a responsibility of the hospital administrator. As the hospital literature on this subject increased, James Hague, the editor of the AHA journal, *Hospitals*, asked me whether I could contribute something. The result was a letter printed in a 1965 issue of *Hospitals*.[1] Twenty years later, I still strongly support the philosophy that the hospital administrator is in a unique position to ensure that there is no discrimination on the basis of race, creed, or color—and beyond this, that the atmosphere of the hospital should be truly color-blind, so that there is no need for special personnel policies.

CORPORATE ORGANIZATION

The other aspect of hospital administration—corporate organization—was of negligible importance from the 1930s to the 1950s. Even the great hospitals of that time had superintendents and directors; their few administrative associates were actually assistants, and the director was thought of primarily as a senior employee paid to operate the hospital. What influence the director did have came from his or her personal stature and personality. This was true even of the giants of that era, such as Washburn and Faxon of MGH, Hamilton of Detroit, Smith of Baltimore, and Mac-Lean. The subject of corporate organization did not even appear upon the agenda of the Society of Medical Administrators and the Medical Administrators Conference until 1972. Gradually, in the 1950s, the hospital administrator began to be accepted as a peer on the board, first as its secretary, later as the executive vice president. In 1962, Johns Hopkins Hospital became one of the first to appoint a CEO (Russell A. Nelson) as president of the hospital. This practice remained unusual for a number of years, but it is now increasingly common.

Partly because of Basil MacLean's indifference to job titles, charts of organization, and formal job descriptions, I paid little attention to these matters until I was faced with the appointment of a new director of nursing at Grace-New Haven. Professor Thomas Spates, who was then professor of personnel administration at Yale University, suggested that I compare the nursing department's size and budget with other departments. This revealed that the tradition of considering the nursing director as another department head, reporting to an assistant director, was ridiculous. Most of the departments had from fifteen to one hundred employees. The director of nursing, however, was responsible for more than six hundred employees and approximately one-third of the hospital budget. The new director of nursing therefore came on as an assistant

1. A. Snoke, "Hospitals and Human Rights," *Hospitals* 39 (April, 1965).

director of the hospital. This was in 1951, and many of my colleagues insisted that they had always considered their directors of nursing in these terms. But it still took years before they formally recognized the position with the appropriate title. Now the director of nursing is a senior administrative officer or senior vice president in most hospitals. Progress has not been very rapid however. *Hospitals* reported in July 1984 that the AHA "is taking steps to restructure its organization to reflect the changing role of the hospital nurse executive." This is being done "in response to consensus by the nursing field and by the AHA's Board of Trustees that the organization representing nurse executives should recognize their role in the executive management team of the hospital."[2]

The chief executive officer is now also the executive vice president or president of the board in most hospitals, while the chairman of the board is a community representative. The emphasis upon titles and upon a more formal, corporate approach is not a matter of self-aggrandizement or higher salaries, but a logical reaction to the changing status of the hospital. Hospitals are big business; frequently they are the major industry in their communities. The CEO has great responsibility from the operational point of view, and to this must be added his or her unique responsibility for the care of the patient and for the role of the hospital in community health. These organizational changes are basically good for the management of the institution. But they lead, of course, to the next logical development—multihospital corporations, consortia, and partnerships. Obvious dangers of this trend are increased emphasis on form and structure, marketing, competition, and the bottom line—with a corresponding loss of interest in the welfare of the patient.

It is essential to the maintenance and survival of the hospital that the CEO carry out effectively the responsibilities of hotel-keeping, fiscal management, personnel administration, corporate reorganization, marketing, and also that he or she maintain good relations with physicians, board, and government. The danger is that these urgent, important demands will overshadow the CEO's basic responsibility for health care in the hospital and in the community. For example, in 1982, a group of sensitive and authoritative health care administrators, all physicians, outlined sixteen points relative to corporate reorganization of hospitals. Fourteen points dealt with legal, fiscal, and organizational factors; only two involved responsibility for patient care.

It is clearly ridiculous to ignore the importance of the institutional operation or the fiscal stability of a hospital in favor of patient care. All are

2. T. Corpuz, "Management Rounds, Support Service," *Hospitals* 58, 14 (July 16, 1984), 82–84.

important, but the boards and the CEOs of hospitals are having an increasingly difficult time maintaining an even balance. Hospital administration is far more complicated today than in the past and outside influences on the hospital have increased markedly. One prominent hospital administrator recently tried to explain to me why he was leaving a prestigious hospital to go into an allied health service. Things are different now, he said, commenting almost enviously that I had lived during the "Golden Age of hospital administration."

This changed environment also has a bearing on Ray Trussell's answer when I upbraided him for responding so negatively to certain cooperative efforts proposed by Blue Cross and the Greater New York Hospital Association. He has an enviable record for his pioneering efforts, at the Hunterdon Medical Center in Flemington, New Jersey, in employing salaried specialists in the hospital while maintaining close professional relationships with community general practitioners; for his teaching programs in public health at Columbia University; and for his work as commissioner of hospitals of New York City. Dr. Trussell simply said, "Today, I am the CEO of a major New York City hospital, and foremost in my responsibilities is the *survival* of that institution."

When one emphasizes the priority of patient care in today's health world, one runs the risk of being considered a soft-headed "do-gooder." However, I was rather shocked when David Winston, senior vice president for planning of the Voluntary Hospitals of America, was quoted as saying that hospitals can no longer think of themselves as community service organizations if they hope to compete successfully for the shrinking pool of capital funds, and that the idea that health care is not a business should be abandoned.[3] Like me, Rashi Fein also disagreed with the point of view that sees patients as teaching material, a medical practice as a business, and delivering medical care as producing a product—all seen in terms of financial transactions.[4] I am not sure that these two men would find themselves so far apart if they tried to develop an overall health policy, but their words, echoed elsewhere, illustrate the problems we face in developing future health care policies.

RESPONSIBILITY FOR CARE OF PEOPLE

I challenge the assumption that care of people and community service must conflict with business. I believe they can be reconciled, that concern

3. D. Winston, "Hospitals Must Think as Businesses to Compete for Capital," quoted in AHA *Hospital Week*, February 10, 1984.

4. R. Fein, "What Is Wrong with the Language of Medicine?" *New England Journal of Medicine*, 58 (1982), 863–64.

with the business aspects of the hospital or of the health system does not have to destroy concern for the people that the business is supposed to serve. Others share my view: Thomas Matherlee emphasized the role of caring in his inaugural address as chairman of the AHA Board of Trustees in January, 1984, and Robert Cunningham pointed out the need to preserve the caring tradition among physicians in spite of the present trend toward corporate organization for health care.[5]

Accepting the importance of the many pragmatic administrative aspects of operating a hospital, I therefore return to my basic thesis that the hospital administrator's primary responsibility is the care of the patient. There are those, of course, who will question this broad statement, because it is unusual for the hospital administrator to be concerned with individual patients. But it is unrealistic to expect that total responsibility for the care of patients can be assumed by physicians or nurses. Nor can this responsibility be carried out by members of the hospital board, no matter how interested or sensitive they may be. Proper care of patients today is a highly complex, multidisciplinary activity, and each group contributing to it has its own interests and priorities. The CEO of the hospital is the only person who can see the overall picture and wield the authority to bring the factions together with the goal of providing this care.

The administrator of a hospital has several assets that can be used to improve patient care in both the hospital and the community. The first is the influence and authority that goes with the position of administrative officer in a major business institution. As the employer of a large number of nursing personnel, I was obviously interested in education and recruitment. In 1940 I stimulated the Department of Vocational Education in the city of Rochester to start one of the first schools of practical nursing in New York State. I learned that the Rochester Board of Education wanted to diversify the vocational curriculum, and I was also aware of the need in our hospital for people with more training than a nurses' aide, but less than a graduate nurse. Knowing that my chief would support me, I offered the SMH as a sponsor and training area. The experience encouraged me to help initiate a state-supported training program for licensed practical nurses (LPNS) when I came to Connecticut.

Shortly after I came to New Haven, the hospital's dietitian was retiring, and I had to search for a replacement. An administrator in Wisconsin highly recommended Doris Johnson, one of the few Ph.D.s in dietetics at that time. We made a deal—she would reorganize the dietary

5. R. Cunningham, "Preserving a Caring Tradition," *Hospitals* 57, 17 (September 1, 1984), 85–88.

department, and incidentally save several hundred thousand dollars a year by combining kitchens and food services, and I would help her start a dietary internship and residency program in the hospital. The twenty-fifth anniversary of the dietary program took place in 1984, with dietitians from all over the country returning to express their appreciation to Dr. Johnson.

A second asset available to the hospital administrator is his exposure to programs and problems in health care throughout the hospital and community and his ability, as a result of his position, to effect change in these areas. As the assistant director of SMH in the early 1940s, I helped the first black woman gain admittance to the Strong Memorial Hospital School of Nursing.

I was also able to discuss with the dean and professor of pathology, George H. Whipple, the high incidence of probable tuberculosis infection among first- and second-year medical students. Bolstered by the research of Gordon Meade, an assistant to Dr. MacLean, I had the temerity to suggest to this Nobel laureate that the infections might be due to his department's techniques in the gross pathology programs and in handling autopsies of patients with tuberculosis. Changes in procedures, more careful attention to the cleaning and sterilization of the autopsy areas, and recognition that tuberculous tissue must be handled carefully resulted in a marked decrease in cases of tuberculosis among the medical students. It is obvious that my position in hospital administration gave me authority and influence that I would not have had as a junior clinician.

Another more dramatic clinical incident, which occurred in Rochester in 1941, demonstrates the value of the hospital administrator's willingness to mobilize services for an experimental technique. Sister Kenny had come from Australia with her new ideas for the treatment of polio. Although she had found a sympathetic base of operations in Minnesota, she was still regarded skeptically by most physicians. According to my friends in Minnesota, she did not help her cause by her abrasive and uncompromising attitude. And, while the results of her method of therapy gained grudging acceptance, her scientific explanations were rather thin. Nevertheless, her ideas attracted national attention. Plato Schwartz, professor of orthopedics at the University of Rochester, went to New York City to attend a conference on her new ideas.

While the orthopedist was in New York City, the seven-year-old son of the hospital maintenance chief was admitted with complete paralysis of an arm and leg caused by polio. He was treated conventionally with casts to prevent abnormal contractures. When Dr. Schwartz returned from the conference, I said that, if he wished to try Sister Kenny's new therapy out on the boy, the hospital would stand behind him. We also helped persuade the family to agree to the then revolutionary therapy.

By that afternoon, the nursing and physical therapy departments had rigged up a mechanism for heating and wringing out towels and blankets for compresses, the casts were off, and passive movement of the limbs had begun. A few weeks later, the boy left the hospital walking on two nearly normal legs and with an arm that was not withered from inaction.

A third asset of the hospital administrator is the ability to implement staff suggestions that cut across many lines of authority and custom. I am particularly proud of my part in developing the rooming-in program in the obstetrical unit of Grace-New Haven. A pediatrician, a nursing instructor, and an obstetrician planned the experimental unit. It had no counterpart in this country, although it was common in many other countries to keep the newborn infant at the mother's bedside. To develop such a unit in New Haven required adjustment to the standardization program of the American College of Surgeons and to the licensing requirements of the Connecticut State Health Department. To my surprise, the program was vehemently opposed by many other pediatricians and obstetricians in the hospital, as well as by the city director of health, himself a pediatrician. Having listened to all objections, I approved the necessary changes in physical structure, staffing patterns, and visiting regulations and I convinced the licensing and accrediting agencies that the experimental program was worth trying. It was the forerunner of similar rooming-in programs throughout the United States.[6]

The concept of rooming-in opened the door to the subsequent development of natural childbirth, the nurse-midwife program at the Yale School of Nursing, prenatal classes for fathers and mothers, attendance of fathers in the delivery room, and the homelike atmosphere in today's delivery suites. If the hospital administrator had not approved—and, indeed, fought for—the rooming-in unit, these programs might have been delayed for years in New Haven. The administrator does not have to be all-knowing. But if he or she is interested in people care and has the ability to listen, learn, and then to act, he or she has a unique opportunity to bring about changes which, with luck, will lead to progress.

A similar improvement in patient care resulted from a request by pediatrician Louis Gluck that I look at the unit for premature infants that we had carefully planned and built a few years earlier at Grace-New

6. A. Snoke, "A Hospital Rooming-In Unit for Newborns and Mother," *Stanford Medical Bulletin* 6, 1 (1948), 143–148; A. Snoke, "Rooming-In and Natural Childbirth in a General Hospital," *Modern Hospital* 71, 3 (1951), 98–110.

Haven. He wanted to expand the facilities to care not only for premature babies but for all newborn infants who might be in need of skilled, intensive care. Together with our nursing supervisors we planned and made the necessary changes in the existing premature nursing unit to meet Dr. Gluck's and the nurses' needs in caring for the acutely ill infants.

Another example of this type of administrative intervention occurred in 1946, when James Rowland Angell, a former president of Yale, was admitted with pneumonia. Wanting to meet him, I went to the patient care division. To my amazement, he was occupying a room in the hospital's Isolation Pavilion. The Pavilion, built around 1920, was known as the Pest House. Patients with tuberculosis, strep throats, pneumonias, and other infections were automatically lodged there in accommodations that were primitive by any standards. Mr. Angell was perfectly satisfied and doing well, but I could see no justification for anyone's being cared for in such surroundings. I told the chairman of the Department of Medicine and the dean of the Medical School, Francis Blake, of Mr. Angell's admission to the Isolation Pavilion. I asked him whether it was really necessary to segregate patients with fever or infection rather than admitting them to ordinary facilities and taking special precautions for those with infectious disease. Dr. Blake, a national authority on infectious disease, recognized the absurdity of the rule, but it had never been changed. We brought up the subject at the next medical board meeting and we changed the admitting policy immediately. In the meantime, Mr. Angell had recovered and gone home. I don't think he ever knew what he had accomplished by his visit.

In the sensitive area of staff and physician schedules, the hospital administrator's authority is especially useful in effecting change. In the late 1940s visiting hours at Grace-New Haven totaled only three hours a day, unless the patient was on the critical list. A few hospitals were experimenting with free visiting from 10:00 A.M. to 8:30 P.M. (with a limit of two visitors at a time), and I asked several members of the nursing staff to visit these Boston hospitals and evaluate the results. They endorsed the concept. But then came the job of rearranging schedules. Virtually every service department in the hospital was sympathetic to the new visiting hours, but they also did not want to have to change their schedules. The changes were really not a matter of great complexity, but it soon became obvious that an overall authority was necessary both to propose the idea and to see that it was implemented. I did it, and a much more convenient visiting schedule for patients and their families resulted. A related, but more difficult task involved patients' complaints about being awakened at 5:30 or 6:00 A.M. to have their temperatures taken and then having to wait several hours for breakfast and for the doctors' rounds. Altering this time-honored procedure required the hospital administrator's authority because it involved nursing, dietary, and housekeeping staff as well as the physicians' scheduled rounds. I persisted, and the result was a step toward a more natural environment for patients.

I was reminded of a third such incident by a fellow patient when I was convalescing from a coronary in 1983. Years earlier, she said, the hospital clinic had the custom of placing a large black bar on the ID cards of welfare patients. She was then working at the local Legal Aid office, and she wrote to me asking if it were necessary to so stigmatize the welfare patients. I inquired of the clinic staff and found no reason for it other than ancient usage. Two weeks later, I wrote to her that the custom had been discontinued.

RECONCILING CORPORATE ORGANIZATION AND PATIENT CARE

Hospitals are legally and morally responsible for the care of patients, and the board and its CEO must develop a comprehensive structure and system to carry out this responsibility. The CEO can delegate experts to deal with operational and fiscal matters; the medical, nursing, and social service staff can take care of individual patients; but he or she is the only person who is in the position to see these activities as a whole and who has the authority to bring these groups together to ensure the best possible care. This fact should be uppermost in the minds of the board of a hospital or health corporation when it chooses a CEO. It should also be emphasized in educational programs designed for health care administrators and should be particularly considered as corporate health organizations grow in numbers and diversity.

Basil MacLean could very well have added the terms *corporate manager* and *strategic planner* to inn-keeper and bookkeeper if he were talking to the AHA in 1984 instead of 1939. A 1984 study by the Arthur Andersen and Co. and the American College of Hospital Administrators (ACHA) indicates a shift in administrative priorities;[7] strategic planning is expected to top the priority list in 1995; horizontal, multihospital corporations are expected to increase in an effort to improve financial stability; and the 1984 AHA House of Delegates has proposed new methods of reimbursement. All indicate that the leaders of the health industry are preoccupied with business matters. J. Alexander McMahon, in his presidential speech to the house of Delegates, almost seemed like a voice crying in the wilder-

7. Arthur Andersen and Co. and the American College of Hospital Administrators, "Health Care in the 1990s: Trends and Strategies," 1984.

ness when he reminded the House of their responsibility for the indigent and aged, for ethics and quality.

As they incorporate either horizontally or vertically, many hospitals will face the problem of how their various boards and administrative officers will continue to meet the legal and moral responsibilities for the care of the patient. My board and I faced no such problem—our respective responsibilities were clear and our means of monitoring performance were directly at hand. It will, however, prove a major challenge to the newly organized corporate hospitals and health care organizations. The CEO and his administrative and medical associates can function efficiently at the local level, but the question remains whether upper-echelon corporate administrators and boards can develop a truly perceptive and authoritative approach to quality review and control. Carrying out this responsibility will become even more difficult as multilevel corporations combine nonprofit and profit divisions and the balance sheet becomes the measure of success or failure. They might perhaps be politely needled by being given a picture of the little statue *Discharged Cured*.

2

Education and Training of the Hospital and Health Administrator

Important to any discussion of the hospital administrator's responsibilities is the matter of his or her education and training. The central debate on this topic has not changed since I entered the field in 1937. Should the education be designed to produce a business or corporate manager or a professional health administrator fundamentally concerned with the total care of the patient? Obviously, there is no sharp separation between these two types, yet educators and administrators have debated for forty years over how to train people to manage increasingly expensive and complex institutions whose primary responsibility is—or should be—the care of people.

Education of hospital administrators—in keeping with their status— was a low priority in the 1930s. Relatively few leaders in the field extended their vision beyond the hospital and believed that care of patients should be as important to the hospital administrator as accounting and hotel-keeping. At that time, most executives advanced from other positions in the hospital; they were directors of nursing, purchasing agents, accountants, or engineers, matrons, and superintendents. One hospital superintendent had the title of "warden." Probably because the hospital was so dominated by the physician, many of the great metropolitan and teaching institutions had physicians as their chief executive officers, and they ruled the hospital world for many years. Although the first six presidents of the American Hospital Association (1899–1904) were nonmedical, thirty-two of the next forty-two presidents (up to 1946) were physicians. So were ten of the next twenty-three (up to 1969). There have been none since.

The relative merits of the physician and nonphysician hospital administrator were still being argued as late as 1982. It is a silly debate. An M.D. degree does not confer administrative skill or common sense any more than a degree from a school of business gives its holder administrative competence, the ability to handle people and maintain budgets, or concern for people's welfare. The hospital or health care administrator is a professional and specialist in his or her own right, whether an M.D. or not. A medical degree does not guarantee an administrator's concern for or influence in the care of patients.

A final comment on physicians as hospital administrators: I doubt that anyone can continue to function as a practicing physician in the hospital of which he is the CEO. Even though this is a common custom in many parts of the world, I have always questioned its wisdom, because of the possibility of conflict of interest and a skewed sense of responsibility and authority. In addition, one person cannot keep up to date professionally and function adequately in both positions. When I started as an assistant director in administration at Strong Memorial Hospital, I was determined to continue with my research and teaching in pediatrics. After two years, however, I gave up pediatrics, because the resident staff and the senior students were more up to date on my clinical specialty than I. When Richard Weinerman came to New Haven to head the Medical Center's Ambulatory Services Program, he insisted that he would continue in cardiology. But he soon found that he could not do justice to both administrative and clinical responsibilities, and he gave up cardiology. I have always wondered why psychiatrists believe they are exceptions and continue to be clinicians as well as administrators of mental hospitals.

The only advantage I saw to having an M.D. degree as a hospital administrator was that it was easier for me to tell a doctor to go to hell, or, to put it more mildly, that I thought his opinion was stupid. Many of my nonmedical colleagues agreed with my attitude but frequently added, "But you can say what you think because you are a doctor." But, while conversations with my professional colleagues may have been less inhibited, I never believed that my administrative judgment was better because of my M.D. degree—and neither did anyone else.

The first formal graduate program in hospital administration was started in 1934 with a grant from the Rosenwald Fund to Michael M. Davis, a professor in the Graduate School of Business at the University of Chicago. After the first year, Arthur Bachmeyer and, later, Ray Brown took over the program as part of their responsibilities as CEOs of the university hospitals and clinics. The program later became an integral part of the graduate school of business, with a full-time faculty.

The Chicago program stimulated graduate training and research in hospital administration, and a new era emerged. Chicago turned out many well-trained and highly motivated individuals. The Kellogg Foundation both supported the Chicago program for a number of years and financed or encouraged similar programs at the schools of public health at Columbia, Yale, Minnesota, Toronto, Pittsburgh, and the University of California, as well as in schools of business administration at Michigan and Northwestern. Programs were also started in schools of medicine in St. Louis (Washington University and St. Louis University) and Iowa.

I had the responsibility of forming the program at Yale in 1946–1947. In 1946, before I moved to New Haven, I happened to have breakfast with Graham Davis, a senior official at the Kellogg Foundation, at an AHA function. He congratulated me on my new appointment and said that the foundation had hoped to finance a program of hospital administration in the School of Public Health at Yale, but Yale had not seemed interested, so they had decided to approach Harvard.

I had heard nothing of this, but I solemnly assured Mr. Davis that there must have been a breakdown in communications, for Yale was very excited about the potential program. I suggested that he call the chairman of the School of Public Health, Ira Hiscock. As soon as breakfast was over, I hurriedly telephoned Dr. Hiscock, who, as I expected, knew nothing of the offer. Mr. Davis called him later that morning; he responded with enthusiasm; and Kellogg made the grant to Yale.

A major challenge to many programs' approaches to the teaching of hospital administration came in 1954, with the release of the report of the Commission on University Education in Hospital Administration (the Olsen Report).[1] Today, it retains an air of Alice-in-Wonderland unreality, but it served to stimulate more definitive thinking on the nature of education and training for the hospital administrator, and after more than twenty-five years it still described quite accurately many of the problems confronting hospitals, society, and the hospital CEO. Unfortunately, its recommendations were too rigid, as if it were describing a military cadet or the typical corporate executive as seen in a *New Yorker* cartoon. They seemed completely inconsistent with the report's excellent description of the administrator's responsibilities.

- The program should be located in a university school of business.
- The age limits should be fixed at twenty-one to twenty-seven.
- The prerequisites for admission should include undergraduate courses in

1. "Commission on University Education in Hospital Administration," published by the American Council on Education, Washington, D.C., 1954.

accounting, statistics, principles of administration, personnel administration, finance, marketing, business law, and general business conditions.
• Training in professional nursing or medicine would not be of value in advanced work in hospital administration.

There was considerable disagreement (including mine) with the conclusion and recommendations of the Commission Report. I maintained that hospital administration was a profession, not a business, and that it involved the formation of a community health center that should include physicians, nursing groups, the community health department, and other health agencies.[2] Even then, I was emphasizing social as well as health needs and pointing out that the hospital administrator should be a health care administrator. Those disagreeing with the majority report (apparently, the vote was almost evenly split) agreed that expertise in management and pragmatic operation were essential, and that philosophy and ideals were useless without the proper organizational structure and adequate personnel to support them. The question was how best to achieve the several objectives. I came out of the debate with three basic convictions. The first was a strengthened belief that the hospital administrator should also be a health care administrator and should feel responsible for the quality of care given to patients. The atmosphere of the educational environment and the attitudes of the faculty and students seemed important in this regard. Although I personally favor a school of public health as the sponsor of the program, it does not matter where it is, so long as it orients the student toward the unique requirements of effective people care.

The second was the obvious point that formal graduate education at a university, leading to a master's degree or a doctorate, is crucial. Regardless of an individual's experience, age, or competence, the advanced degree should be a requirement for obtaining an initial position—or for promotion. And my third conviction was that education in this field cannot be considered complete at the end of the several years spent obtaining a degree. Academic courses, theses, computer training, and expertise in statistical analysis, along with active participation in seminars and research projects, merely give the student a background for further education and training. Programs to allow the student to obtain actual administrative experience under supervision, after the degree, are necessary.

At Yale we tried, from the first class in 1947, to make the graduate students feel that they were in a professional environment, directly

2. A. Snoke, "Hospital Administration is a Profession—not a Business," *Modern Hospital* 84, 1 (1955), 61–62, 150.

involved in health care. There were formal lectures and demonstrations for the hospital administration group as well as presentations to the public health students as a whole, but instruction was in seminars whenever possible. Classes were limited to ten or twelve, and students were selected on the basis of maturity and experience—particularly in some aspect of health or social science. Hospital department heads and administration were intimately involved with the clear understanding that the entire hospital and medical center was to be the students' laboratory. As a professor—but not the director of the program—I held a weekly seminar in which I involved the class in administrative problems and decisions. These sessions dealt with problems that I (as an active administrator) was confronting at the moment. The only rule was that our discussions had to be confidential. For the twenty years I led my seminar, confidentiality was never broken.

During one meeting, I asked them how they thought I should deal with a department head whose responsibilities had grown beyond his capacity. At the end of the session I learned to my horror that the class was scheduled for a meeting the next hour with that very individual. They said nothing. Another time, students participated in a two-hour session with me and a former graduate. His hospital's medical staff were refusing to admit patients unless the board fired him. His crime was trying to make the medical staff observe the sanitary procedures that they themselves had established.

Sometimes I opened my mail with the students, so that we could discuss what to do about letters or comment cards that I received. On one of these occasions I received an emergency call from the AHA in Washington, telling me that Wilbur Mills, in consultation with representatives of organized medicine and hospital-based specialties, had decided to shift radiology and pathology from part A (hospital costs) to part B (physician fees) of the Medicare legislation. The students were aware of the potential effects on hospital patients. Subsequently, they were kept up to date on the discussions and correspondence that later developed into the Senate's Douglas Amendment for Medicare.

I suspect the students recognized that our discussions were not only a learning experience for them but a very valuable consultation for me. We often took a vote on what I should do—and when I later reported on what I had actually done and what had happened, I or they sometimes had to eat crow. I have been flattered when, in recent years, a number of my former students—many of whom are now CEOs of major teaching hospitals—have told me that these seminar sessions were one of the most interesting and valuable experiences in their educational program.

As important as I considered the formal, academic program in the university, I regarded the residency and continuing education thereafter as equally, if not more, important. Clement Clay was the first director of the Yale program, and he shared my philosophy. He spent as much time planning his students' residencies and observing the work of his residency preceptors as he did in organizing the academic program. We were both convinced that a blend of natural maturation, exposure to and explanation of the successes and failures of individuals or programs, and gradually increasing responsibility were essential to developing administrators.

I thought I knew everything at the end of four years of medical school—and I was even more certain of my ability and knowledge after five years of internship and residency. But I found I was continually learning throughout my years in administration. I came to appreciate more and more my ten years of postgraduate education with Basil MacLean, which taught me several crucial aspects of my job:

- I learned to deal on a collegial basis with administrative associates and department heads—particularly when they knew more about the intricacies of a particular subject than I did.
- I was reminded to observe lines of communication and authority. This was always difficult for me. It seemed so easy to let the urge to "run and find out" (the philosophy, as my wife constantly reminded me, of Kipling's mongoose, Rikki Tikki Tavi) cut unfairly across the lines of authority and responsibility of my associates.
- I learned to delegate responsibility and then back up my associates if a mistake was made—if I wanted to disagree, I had to do it in private.
- I kept aware of the daily activities of patient care, for only in this way could my associates and I keep track of what was happening to the patients who were our responsibility. The picture of the little statue *Discharged Cured* was the subject of a seminar with the class every year. Its philosophy is at least as important as the balance sheet.

A final comment should be made regarding education in the health field. Given the size and complexity of the health industry (it is about the third largest in the nation) and the number of people it employs, it is natural to expect educational institutions to provide expanded opportunities for study in this field. But they must avoid the danger of overproducing undergraduate majors in health care and hospital administration, as well as in planning, financing, budgeting, personnel management, public relations, marketing, and education in these areas. The program may be academically sound, but few positions are available for people with only a bachelor's degree. The college graduate will either end up in a low-level job or have to continue for a master's degree. In addition, there is an ever-increasing danger that these graduates will immediately accept positions in health agencies or in some minor political arenas, where they will become instant authorities because of their positions but without the benefit of knowledge or experience. With government regulation and control increasing, this lack of expertise may prove to be a major problem for the health care administrator.

3

The Governing Board

Whenever hospital administrators were asked to suggest subjects for seminars or conferences, problems related to the governing board and to the medical staff always seemed to top the lists. Today, the agendas for such meetings include topics hardly dreamed of two decades ago, from corporate reorganization and strategic planning to plain survival. Yet relations with physicians and trustees continue to be vital subjects for consideration.

The relationship of the administrator to the hospital board and the board's representation and responsibilities have changed markedly over the years. When I began in hospital administration, the voluntary hospital board was usually made up of people with social and philanthropic prestige and a strong sense of obligation. They played major roles in the early growth of community hospitals and in the great private university hospitals. Administrators were hired hands. Expertise in fiscal matters and operations, as well as the power to shape overall policy, belonged to the board—with due deference to the medical staff. Difficulties began to arise when the business of hospitals became more complex, when hospitals were recognized as specialized institutions and more administrators came armed with graduate degrees in hospital and health-care administration. These administrators attracted associates who were experts in hospital operation. As might be expected, conflict arose between administrators and members of the hospital boards, who were often specialists in their own jobs and who expected to assume substantial authority in the hospital.

Regardless of the potential problems inherent in the independent board, its value was so clear that even the individualistic administrator Basil MacLean secured a board for Strong Memorial Hospital. It was set up as a separate entity within the University of Rochester Board of

22

Trustees, because Dr. MacLean saw the need for an identifiable community body responsible for hospital operations. Over the years, such boards have been established in a number of university teaching hospitals, remaining separate from the university trustees.

RESPONSIBILITY

There is no question of the importance of the hospital board. It is legally and morally responsible for everything that happens in the hospital and answerable to the community and to the patients for the caliber of the health practitioners to whom it gives hospital privileges and for the care they provide. It now can be sued for malpractice. The board is also responsible for the fiscal viability of the institution and for long-range planning, public relations, and reputation.

In the old, relatively uncomplicated days, doctors cared for sick people, the superintendent ran the institution, and the board concerned itself with the hospital's fiscal health, amenities, gifts, and public relations. Today, as administrators have become professional and the medical staff has become more organized and collectively responsible, the board has become more aware of its broadened responsibility for a people-oriented institution.

This new awareness of collective responsibility has come slowly to most hospitals, and it is now being further complicated by a new trend—the formation of multihospital corporations (both profit and nonprofit), and even super-corporations involving other business enterprises. The trend toward multihospital and health-system corporations will be discussed further in chapter 7, but it is important to emphasize here that the hospital patient, the potential hospital patient, and the community deserve a certain basic assurance. The hospital to which they are admitted must not only be legally and morally responsible for their care, but this responsibility must be clearly defined and accepted by the hospital board, the administrator, and the medical staff.

Admittedly, it is an oversimplification merely to say that the board is responsible for everything that happens in the hospital. What does this mean, and how can the board carry out its responsibilities? Many years ago, the chairman of Otis Elevator, LeRoy A. Petersen, who served with me on the Carrier Corporation board, outlined to me his concept of the primary responsibilities of a board as we were trying to solve a sensitive personality problem in Carrier's senior administrative hierarchy. Mr. Petersen listed three basic responsibilities for the board:

1. To set the objectives and policies of the corporation;
2. To select a chief executive officer to carry them out; and
3. To keep out of his administrative hair.

I have tried over the years to apply these guidelines to the hospital industry. It seems appropriate, but the product is not a motor or an elevator, but something far more complex—the well-being of a human being in the context of his or her family and community. Most board members have no trouble with the traditional fiduciary and operational responsibilities expected of them. On the hospital board, however, they must also devise means to ensure that an elusive but essential product—high-quality care for the patients—is delivered. The explosive expansion in medical knowledge and techniques, the growing range and complexity of services offered by the hospital, and the increasing cost of these services to the patient and the community make this responsibility increasingly difficult to carry out.

Part of the answer is the employment of a professional hospital administrator. Having chosen one, the board must help him or her develop the most effective management and organization to provide high quality care. The medical staff must also be appropriately organized to be able to provide satisfactory professional leadership and services.

REPRESENTATION

One answer to broadening problems is to broaden representation on the board. This trend, however, has developed slowly. The board in New Haven in 1946 was a typical example of the traditional community hospital board. It included many local CEOs in business, banking and utilities, and several prominent lawyers. I had great difficulty convincing them that anyone besides Anglo-Saxon, Republican businessmen or lawyers should be on the board. They were proud, however, when they took the first step toward a broadened representation by electing a Democratic Jewish banker. Labor representatives, women, and members of minority groups came later. It took me and my associates years to realize that this expansion of representation was not merely a gesture toward participatory democracy, but a valuable asset. As other voices and opinions were heard in board meetings, we learned of differing needs and points of view.

Physicians on the Board

Doctors on the hospital board present a sensitive problem of representation. Specific questions that need to be addressed by any board are:

Should the medical staff be represented on the governing board? If so, what is the proper relationship of the physician board member to his or her staff, to the rest of the board, and to the administrator? During the 1930s and 1940s, to question the wisdom of having doctors on the hospital board of directors was very difficult. The doctors dominated the hospital. The board members were comfortable controlling its institutional and fiscal operations but felt no one but the doctor could speak professionally regarding the care of the patients. Many hospitals had been started by doctors, and some were completely dominated by one or two senior physicians who had built the institution into a powerful force in the community.

However, as hospitals grew in size and complexity, more broadly educated and experienced people were required to run them. Boards recognized that, if these administrators were to function effectively, they must be given full support—even over the potential opposition of physicians. Physicians were of great value on the board if they functioned as advisors. But they could cause disaster if they saw themselves as spokespersons for the medical staff. The situation was often made worse if the physician board members were elected by their associates. And an added problem was often that, even if physicians did not expect special respect, they were regarded by lay board members as superior authorities in the health world because they were doctors. (The phrase "M-Deity" may be a bit unfair, but it does reflect certain realities.) Thus doctors' comments on questions before hospital boards frequently carried more weight than they deserved.

In spite of these problems, I believe that the judgment and advice of the medical staff is essential to the effective administration of a hospital. Therefore, I discussed with the medical board the possibility that its chairman or chief of staff might join or at least meet with the hospital's governing board. We concluded, however, that, given the physician's unique position in the hospital hierarchy, there might be more efficient and less dangerous means of conveying medical staff opinions to the board. Our solution was the joint conference committee, which included members of the board, the administration, and the medical staff. The committee explored policy and administrative issues in detail. If necessary for a special discussion, medical staff representation on the board was arranged. However, the committee turned out to provide the best organizational framework for communication, advice, and action.

Both medical staff leaders and hospital board members recognize another important factor in physician trusteeship: the doctor's unique personal influence with individual members of the board. The personal physicians of most board members and their families are members of the hospital's medical staff. Opinion can also be sought or offered through social contacts. Although these outside influences were stronger in the early days of professional hospital administration, they can still make the hospital CEO's job more difficult than that of other executives. The present trend to make CEOS formal members of the board helps to alleviate this problem. My answer to the question whether a physician can be on a hospital board has always been "of course—depending on the physician." Many fine hospitals have physicians on their governing boards. But I do feel that the alternative we developed was a preferable mechanism for carrying out our mutual objectives.

MEDICAL PRIVILEGES AND DISCIPLINE

The legal and moral responsibility of the hospital board for patient care implies a need to monitor the quality of the care rendered by physicians. The role of the hospital board in disciplining members of the medical staff is, however, seldom discussed. (This subject will be pursued further in the chapter on medical staff.)

When someone seeks a reliable physician, he or she often asks where a doctor has hospital privileges. Since the hospital board grants these privileges, the public assumes that the doctor's training and competence has been professionally reviewed before he or she is allowed to join the staff. Because it is difficult for a lay board or a CEO to make professional judgments, a medical staff organization is set up, the leaders of which make recommendations to the board for appointments and privileges. A well-organized medical staff with qualified leaders in the various specialties can and should screen applicants and evaluate the performance of the medical staff. But what is to be done when a physician's professional performance—because of illness, alcohol, drugs, or age—falls below standard? In such a case, the hospital board has a special responsibility in medical discipline and a unique power to monitor the quality of care in the voluntary hospitals. Through participation on medical and joint conference committees, lay board members can exert a strong positive influence during consideration of serious problems in physicians' practice or conduct. The lay member's presence in such discussions helps the medical staff leaders judge their associates objectively. Working together, both physicians and laypeople realize that one does not have to be a doctor to judge a physician's character, honesty, and dependability.

MEDDLER'S ITCH

Otis Elevator's Mr. Petersen's insistence that the board stay out of the CEO's hair is probably even more important in the hospital than in industry. This philosophy is piously and frequently endorsed by hospital trustees, even as they blithely ignore it. It isn't that they don't know better—many are CEOs of their own corporations and would never tolerate the board's interference in their own internal administration. Nevertheless, many of them seem to check their administrative experience at the door when they enter the hospital boardroom. I received an extensive education in these problems as former students and assistants came to me for advice over the years.

I still recall the frustration of the administrator of a major teaching institution in Pittsburgh, whose board seemed to include the head of every prestigious corporation or foundation in the area. But the board continually acceded to ridiculous arrangements with the medical staff and the university, arrangements which put the administrator in an impossible situation. In doing so, they acted completely contrary to the administrative principles they insisted upon in their own corporations. Another administrator told me in despair of the gentle but persistent efforts of one senior board member to take over the hospital's business affairs. I came in as a consultant and found an example of an all-too-common situation. The board member was retired and wished—with the best of intentions—to assume the same responsibilities in the hospital that he had held in his own corporation. This meant an office in the hospital and control of the business department—not as an assistant to the administrator, but as a board member. He honestly believed he would be helping—while, incidentally, keeping himself occupied during his retirement. This is an example of what Basil MacLean called "meddler's itch," and it is most virulent when the board member has an office in the hospital. In this situation, I suggested two alternatives: persuade the board member to remain one, or fire the administrator. The board accepted the first recommendation.

"Meddler's itch" occasionally results from corporate handling of an executive who is becoming increasingly ineffective. Instead of arranging for early retirement, the corporation cuts away his or her responsibilities and staff and then assigns the official to represent the company in the community. Thus, many community institutions and agencies find such an individual on their board, eager to fill up his or her empty hours by meddling in the operational affairs of the hospital or agency. This is a touchy situation, but the hospital should not be used by corporations as a solution to their personnel problems.

THE CEO

In determining and carrying out policy it is of course too easy to say—as I
have done—that the board decides on the policy and the CEO executes it.
The hospital and the board are not getting their money's worth under
such an arrangement. If the CEO's abilities are to be fully utilized, then he
or she must also be a consultant to the board and, as such, should play an
important role in the determination of policy.

Mutual confidence is essential to hospital management. No CEO is as
expert in a particular field as are those who work in it, but he or she has
the responsibility of administration. Friendly, loyal, and supportive relations with subordinates and partnership with board members preserve
the integrity of the top position while taking advantage of everyone's
abilities and knowledge.

I found that the same techniques I used as a consultant—offering
information, alternative options, and specific recommendations—were
appropriate in dealing with my own board. I made every effort to present
all the facts and see all the alternatives considered. I then offered my own
recommendations and the reasons for them. The board made the final
decision. If it was not what I had recommended, I at least knew that the
decision had been informed. It was then my responsibility to implement
the decision.

I functioned the same way with my administrative assistants and
department heads. They usually knew more about their own fields than I
did, so I was careful to obtain from them not only information but advice
as well. Sometimes they did not agree with my final decision, just as I did
not always agree with the hospital board's decisions. Sometimes they
argued with me and tried to change the decision, just as I tried to change
the board members' minds. But, in the meantime, we implemented the
policy.

My work with the staff and with the board in developing policies and
planning for the future helped crystallize my attitude toward the traditional retirement age of sixty-five for the CEO. Admittedly, some individuals get old faster and should retire much earlier—and others are
extremely effective at seventy-five. However, I found that combined with
my daily management responsibilities was a constant preoccupation with
the hospital's future relationship to the medical school, the university,
and the community. At forty-five or fifty, I wondered how much of this
long-range vision I would retain at the age of sixty-five. I have always tried
to look ahead, but I was also suspicious enough of myself to encourage
younger administrative associates and younger members of the board to
continue to ask themselves how we could do better and how best to

prepare for the future. I planned to fire myself as CEO at sixty-five or sixty-eight years of age.

CONTRIBUTIONS OF THE HOSPITAL BOARD

Up to now, I have discussed the responsibilities of hospital boards in relation to the administration of the hospital. Attention must also be given to the tremendous contributions that board members of voluntary hospitals can make, both to their own institutions and to the local, statewide, and national health care environments.

Private philanthropy has always been taken for granted as a major concern of a hospital board. The philanthropic portion of hospitals' income has been decreasing steadily. Nevertheless, board members continue to exert a degree of influence upon the hospital system unmatched in other industries, and they remain uniquely valuable in obtaining community support. They can also assist the broader voluntary health system when adequately oriented and given a chance.

Connecticut offers excellent examples of the influence of lay hospital trustees on the health field. In 1946, the Connecticut Hospital Association (CHA) was essentially a private men's club and admiration society, with the male administrators meeting for dinner once a month. I helped reorganize the association to include each hospital's administrator and the president of the board. A custom was established whereby the presidency of the association alternated between an administrator and a board member, and there were always several board members (and finally some women) on the CHA board. Basil MacLean had done the same thing with the Rochester Hospital Council ten years earlier, and I had been impressed with the authority and influence the hospital trustees lent to that organization. Many state hospital associations, however, have been laggard in enlisting this resource. (At the risk of sounding snide, I will say that hospital administrators sometimes seem afraid of board members.) But I am told that, due to the closer working relationships of the various state hospital associations, stimulated by the AHA, a number of other states are now realizing the value of an informed group of hospital trustees.

Trustees' involvement in Connecticut state hospitals has been far-reaching. In 1948–49, we persuaded the governor to set up a special committee on hospital reimbursement. This was a major step forward: the informed hospital trustees on the CHA board played a major role in passing legislation considered revolutionary at the time. It will be discussed in detail in chapter 8. The hospital trustees also played an important role in the formation, in 1965, of the independent, statewide Connecticut Hospital Planning Commission (separate from the CHA), the first of its kind in the country. The majority of its members, including the officers, were hospital trustees. An example of their statesmanship occurred when the CHPC staff recommended disapproval of the planning applications of the Waterbury and Bristol hospitals. Although the presidents of the two hospital boards were also the president and vice president of the planning commission, they voted to support the staff's recommendation.

Although at times I was discouraged with my board's preoccupation with the balance sheet, enough interest was shown in the welfare of patients to keep me aware of its potential power. One of the most memorable examples of this power occurred at a board meeting in the early 1960s, when I introduced the subject of pregnancies among unmarried teenagers. An administrative associate, Herbert Paris, had earlier brought Philip Sarrel to see me because of his work with pregnant teenagers.[1] Dr. Sarrel was an OB-GYN resident and had conducted a study of 100 unmarried girls aged twelve to seventeen. The girls had had 340 pregnancies. Dr. Sarrel worked closely with them and their families and, one year later, 94 percent had not become pregnant again. I considered this remarkable. Education and contraception were important factors, but the personal attention and involvement of the doctor was crucial. During the conversation I idly asked what happened with the girls' education after they became pregnant. Dr. Sarrel told me that Hartford and other cities were developing constructive programs to deal with the problem, but the boards of education in New Haven and the surrounding towns were merely punitive. When an unmarried schoolgirl became pregnant, out she went.

I arranged for Mr. Paris and Dr. Sarrel to come to the next board meeting, where Dr. Sarrel again described his study. The board was fascinated by his report and impressed with the doctor himself as he described a twelve-year-old whose only concept of her pregnancy was that she was going to get a doll. During the discussion, I "innocently" asked Dr. Sarrel about the girls' education. He described the attitude of the New Haven Board of Education. I turned to Arnon Thomas, the hospital's counsel, and asked him why the hell his law partner, who was chairman of the New Haven Board of Education, did not do something about it. Mr. Thomas muttered that he was shocked and would talk to his

1. P. M. Sarrell, "The University Hospital and the Teenage Mother," *American Journal of Public Health* 57, 8 (1967), 1308; P. M. Sarrell, "The Young Unwed Mother—A Study of 100 Cases with Five Year Follow-up," *American Journal of Obstetrics and Gynecology* 95, 5 (1966), 722.

partner the next morning. I know nothing of their conversation or the later discussions of the Board of Education, but within a few months pregnant schoolgirls in New Haven were able to continue their education.

The voluntary hospital, with its responsible community board of directors, has been a major factor in the development of the American health system. Recognizing that the health world will continue to change, undoubtedly becoming more complex and costly as diagnostic and treatment procedures multiply, the acute-care hospital will continue to be of fundamental importance. As the interrelationship of health and social services becomes more evident, there will be an even greater need to integrate our human service resources to avoid fragmentation and diffusion of responsibility. The role of the hospital and its governance will continue to be of vital importance; responsibility must be more clearly defined at the local level. If the legitimate needs of the public are not met, government intervention is possible. I am afraid both potential developments—government control, with its politicians and bureaucrats, and the multilayer corporate environment, preoccupied with organization and profits—will place the welfare of the patient at the remotest end of the health care spectrum. The CEO can be fired by the supercorporation, and politicians and bureaucrats can dismiss hospital administrators and doctors as special pleaders. A local, representative hospital board—as my experience in Connecticut showed me—can be a powerful influence in preserving consideration of the patient.

4

The Medical Staff

As has been noted, problems related to the medical staff and the governing board have always had top priority among hospital administrators.
New Haven in 1946 was no exception. We had the same town-and-gown
problems that had existed in Rochester, with the notable difference that
the University of Rochester owned its hospital and medical school, and
there were five other hospitals in the city. Friction and potential conflict
were intensified in New Haven because the hospital was independent
from Yale and because New Haven had only one other hospital. As a
result, organizational and personal relationships involving the administrator, the governing board, and the individual physicians—both in
private practice and on the medical school faculty—were more sensitive.

These problems never seem to disappear. Almost thirty-five years
later, in 1980, medical staff relationships were the subject to which the
alumni of the University of Toronto School of Hospital Administration
gave top priority at a working conference. (I was invited to give the
keynote speech.) Despite the problems of Diagnostic Related Groups and
financial survival, the American College of Hospital Administrators also
gave top priority to hospital-physician relationships at a 1985 conference.

A battle took place in New Haven in 1980–83 among the Yale-New
Haven Hospital, the Yale Medical School, and a number of community
physicians, who attempted to resolve their differences through the
courts. The issue was relatively clearcut: was access to patient beds as well
as to the associated hospital facilities and services equally available to
university physicians and community doctors? Although the medical
board said yes, some remained skeptical because of what they deemed
arbitrary and inequitable decisions by certain university chiefs of service.

32

Not until the board of trustees produced a clear statement of policy did the three factions, all with their legal representatives, reach a settlement that stated simply: "Access to hospital resources by community surgeons, obstetricians, and gynecologists should be afforded on a fair and non-discriminatory basis without regard to whether such physicians are community physicians or university physicians." The three-year experience with its attendant frustration and expense is an excellent example of the difficulties involved in trying to solve operating and administrative problems through recourse to lawyers and judges. Any solution to problems of patient care, assignment of professional privileges and responsibilities, and working relationships among professionals must depend on the organization, personalities, and particularly the leadership in the hospital's administration and the medical staff.

The fact that administrators and physicians have different points of view is easy to understand. From the time the medical student is first exposed to patients and to clinical medicine, the hospital is his or her domain. The physician takes it for granted that hospital services were his or her due, and that he or she is the boss. The system supports this attitude. A hospital's reputation depends on its doctors—the best-staffed and best-equipped hospital is still only mediocre if the doctors are mediocre. And hospitals' financial stability depends upon the doctors, who decide when and where patients should be hospitalized, what should be done for them there, and when they should be discharged. The physician also plays a major role in determining the atmosphere of the hospital. All this means that it is unrealistic to equate the effect of the doctor on the health care dollar with the percentage of that dollar represented by physician fees. When I first came across such statistics, medical charges were roughly 28 percent and hospital expenses were less than 20 percent. Now the pie charts indicate an impressive reversal, with hospital costs accounting for substantially over 40 percent of health care costs and physician fees about 20 percent. These comparative statistics are relatively meaningless, however, for they do not take into account the physician's influence upon hospital costs. It has been estimated that the physician influences approximately 70–75 percent of the health care expenditures to which hospital costs are a major contributing item.[1] The most unusual feature of the physician-hospital relationship is that the doctor is essentially a private entrepreneur who uses the hospital as he or she sees fit. The doctor's word is—or has been—law in most institutions. However,

1. National Committee for Quality Health Care, "The Physician's Role in Health Care Cost Containment," January, 1983; T. Nesbit, "Report on Conference on Hospitals and Health Maintenance Organizations," *Hospitals* 57, 15 (August 1, 1983), 23.

although he or she has a profound influence upon the hospital's utilization, reputation, and financial stability, in most cases, the doctor is not personally at financial risk.

Although I do not underestimate the influence of physicians or their importance in the field of health care, I never considered relations with them a major problem. Of course there were professional difficulties, but I cannot recall any insoluble ones during the twenty-two years I was in New Haven or during the previous ten years in Rochester. Partly this was due to the organizational framework of the two centers, much of which had been developed before I arrived. But the relative lack of conflict was probably due primarily to the professional and leadership qualities of the physicians' representatives on the medical board and its various committees. I suspect that my placidity with regard to physician relationships had something to do with the fact that I was a physician and came from a family of physicians, and I had married a physician from a family of physicians.

I am proud to be a physician, but I have no delusion of omniscience. Far from automatically conferring common sense, competence, administrative ability, or idealism, the selection and training of doctors combine to skew the doctors' outlook, ego, and patterns of conduct. The doctor's focus is primarily upon the patient, his or her independence, and his or her personal practice. Although many studies have indicated high idealism in first- and second-year medical students, idealism tends to diminish rapidly as the student advances. In fact, the whole educational environment and the huge amount of knowledge that the student must absorb contribute to the doctor's centering attention on the patient in a one-to-one relationship. The longer the training and the greater the responsibility given to the young physician, the greater the emphasis placed on his or her final decision. The student recognizes that, as a doctor, he or she will have to take final responsibility for the care of the patient. The buck stops there.

These responsibilities cannot help but make most physicians individualists. It is thus easy to understand the doctor's self-protective attitude, in which outside influences—particularly nonmedical or administrative ones—are regarded with suspicion lest they interfere with his or her independence of judgment or action or in some way affect his or her reputation. The doctor believes that hospital and patient routines are properly adjusted to his or her needs. Finally, the pocketbook is another sensitive area for many physicians. Frequently they see their independence of action or their relationship with the hospital as affecting their income. This is understandable, but it should not be confused with ethics or professionalism as some medical and specialty societies have done.

MEDICAL STAFF ORGANIZATION

I recall with amusement the reactions of each new class in hospital administration at Yale to my questions, "How should a medical staff be organized? Who should promulgate the medical staff bylaws? How should the medical staff leaders be selected?" The students sometimes found it difficult to act polite when I asked such stupid questions. They invariably answered that the medical staff in any hospital of reasonable size should have departments of medicine, surgery, obstetrics-gynecology, and pediatrics, plus a chief of staff or president; the medical staff as a whole should develop and adopt its own bylaws; and each department should elect its leaders and chiefs of service. They were always shocked when I disagreed. Each year, our discussions ranged from the practical realities in our hospital to medical staff problems that I was encountering in hospitals throughout the country. The situation in New Haven was particularly complicated with an independent hospital, a community board, and a medical staff including the medical school faculty and two sets of community physicians.

As usual, the community board of directors was responsible for all activities in the hospital. The medical staff was obviously essential in the care of patients, but ultimate responsibility and authority remained with the board and was delegated to the CEO.[2] The board, however, had no expertise in medicine, nor could the CEO, whether a doctor or not, be expected to have the competence to direct the care of the individual patient. Thus they depended upon the medical staff to carry out this responsibility. This was done by appointing certain physicians as chiefs of service. The board and I expected these chiefs to function in an administrative as well as a professional capacity in carrying out the patient-care responsibilities of the hospital and guiding their colleagues in this task.

The principle that the chiefs' authority came from their appointment by the board was sometimes challenged. When this happened, I asked the medical staff how they expected me to select the chief dietitian or the chief nurse. Should they be elected by the dietitians or nurses? No one advocated this procedure for dietitians or nurses—but doctors, they believed, were different. I accepted the uniqueness of physicians, but not

2. I was surprised to read recently that the philosophy of giving the hospital board ultimate authority was basic to the operation of the first hospital in the country. This was the Pennsylvania Hospital, founded by a group of laymen, most of them businessmen (and including Benjamin Franklin), in 1755. The managers "consulted the doctors and listened to their requests for changes in the building's interior . . . but . . . they always stood ready to check the doctors' desires if they conflicted with the well-being of the patients. They were the final voice of authority." David Freeman Hawke, "Reflections on a University Hospital—200 Years Ago," paper presented at a symposium at the Yale University School of Medicine in 1984.

with regard to the responsibility of selection. The issue can be explored from another angle. Is the medical board a democratically representative body or an administrative body? My answer was always that, given the responsibilities of the hospital board, the medical board must be an *administrative* body. Many concessions to democracy and representation might be made—as long as the basic authority of the hospital board and the CEO was not impaired.

I also made a clear distinction between the organization and authority of the medical board and the organization of the medical staff. The hospital exists for the community; it cares for the people of the community and it provides a mechanism by which physicians and other health-care practitioners can offer such care. The hospital's management, which must bear these broad responsibilities, cannot be subordinate to any specific group. Its administration can be no more democratic than that of any other business or service institution. This in no way forbade the medical staff to organize as a separate and independent group. The staff's elected officers were valued associates and spokespersons. Their organization was specifically provided for in the hospital bylaws, and their president and immediate past president were automatically members of the medical board.

The chiefs of service were selected only after careful consultation with colleagues. The final appointment, for a specified term, was made after the involvement of a search committee and after an informal poll of the staff involved. Without consultation and consideration, few appointments could have been expected to be successful. In only one case, the staff and the search committee were equally divided between two physicians. The board then chose one on their judgment of his superior administrative ability.

When I came to New Haven, I was fortunate to find that the Grace Hospital board had decided several years earlier that the chiefs of service would be appointed by the board after consultation with the medical staff, not elected by the medical staff. This decision apparently triggered a bitter fight among the representatives of the medical staff, and the advocates of democracy finally left the institution for a neighboring hospital. Later, I appreciated the courage of this community board. In 1946, very few hospitals in Connecticut used the appointment method.

In the 1950s, Meriden, Connecticut, had only one hospital, whose medical staff was evenly divided between two factions, one led by a respected medical statesman for Connecticut and the AMA and the other by another prominent local physician. In the yearly elections, the balance between the factions shifted just enough for new leaders to be elected and the old side thrown out. This flip-flop went on until the groups became so disenchanted with each other that the community became involved and, finally, a second hospital was built. Meriden needed two hospitals like it needed two city halls, but medical politics forced this foolish duplication. In the late 1970s, the Connecticut State Hospital Cost Commission forced the two hospitals to form a joint planning committee to explore the possibility of a merger. A merger was recommended by the committee, but it did not occur because of the same attitudes that had caused the split thirty years earlier. Some gestures toward consolidation have been made, but the two separate hospitals remain in active competition in a region with a population of approximately seventy thousand—a one-hospital area by any standard. The two Meriden hospitals represent an unfortunate and expensive exercise in administrative democracy.

Is it, then, impossible for an elected medical board to function satisfactorily? Of course not. A number of fine hospitals in this country use such an arrangement. My position is the same as in the question of having physicians on the governing board: of course it can work, with the right people. But the issue is whether there is a better method of selection, one that consistently functions to meet the needs of the institution, the medical staff, and the patients. I think appointment is better.

OFFICES

Originally, the community chiefs of service at Grace-New Haven retained private offices in the community and came to the hospital to see patients and to participate in various professional and administrative meetings. These tasks were onerous and time-consuming, and the community chiefs were at a disadvantage. The university chiefs, whose offices were located in the medical center complex, were more readily available to the administration, their colleagues, the residents, and the patients. The medical staff and their chiefs were approached with the suggestion that the hospital provide private offices and conference space for the community chiefs. They accepted the idea, and offices were constructed for the community chiefs of medicine, surgery, and obstetrics-gynecology. (The chief of pediatrics declined because his practice primarily involved ambulatory patients.)

The new arrangements were even more successful than we had hoped. We had agreed initially that the community chiefs would pay rent for their office space. But before the end of the first year it became obvious that the value of their presence in the hospital was far greater than any rental income. From then on they were not asked to pay rent. The effectiveness of this full-time arrangement was an important factor in the decision of the Connecticut Regional Medical Program (CRMP) to promote similar arrangements in other hospitals in the state. Prior to 1966, when CRMP started emphasizing its value, the system was used at only four hospitals in Connecticut. By 1975, thirty hospitals in the state had similar arrangements. Even though CRMP is now defunct, thirty out of thirty-four non-university hospitals in Connecticut continue to follow this practicum for a total of ninety-four positions. The usefulness of this arrangement obviously simplifies the question of election versus appointment.

MEDICAL STAFF BYLAWS

Medical staff bylaws were a subject about which I could never get very excited. Much was boilerplate, and, if the hospital's overall objectives and policies were clear, the bylaws were drafted quite easily. There are only a few things that I feel should be emphasized.

- The standard provision that the ethics of the members of the medical staff should conform to those proposed by the AMA is fine, as long as they relate to an ethical code promulgated by the AMA as of a specific date. Ethics have been too easily confused with economics by some special interest groups, and definitions can change.
- Membership in county, state, or national medical associations should not be a requirement for hospital staff privileges.
- The preparation of the bylaws should be the responsibility of the medical staff, with the clear understanding that the authority for their final adoption rests with the board of directors.
- Specific attention should be given to: the composition and method of appointment of the medical board, its responsibilities, the method of selection of new medical staff officers, and the procedure for withdrawing privileges or disciplining staff members.
- The method for adoption and changes of medical staff bylaws should be clearly defined.

Frequently, bylaws that were drawn up years ago were protective of the existing medical hierarchy, and the method for changing them was either nonexistent or confusing and tortuous. For example, in a large New Jersey hospital, the medical staff bylaws provided for a medical board to meet monthly, but also required that no action be implemented without the approval of the entire medical staff, which only met four times a year. The result was considerable activity but little progress. The bylaws also required that any new physician, no matter how well qualified, had to practice in a subordinate position on the medical staff for a number of years, with a senior staff member assuming responsibility for his hospitalized patients. I pointed out that it was ridiculous for a neurosurgical specialist who had completed five to seven years of residency to have to put up with this type of supervision—and fee-sharing—with a probably less competent or less experienced "sponsor." The senior staff members agreed, but they justified continuation of the practice on the grounds that *they* had had to serve this way to get full privileges. It took the hospital board several years to adjust their bylaws and the medical staff bylaws so as to give full privileges to qualified physicians and to have a representative and authoritative medical board. The result was not popular with a number of the medical staff members, who responded by mounting a boycott of the board president's department store.

QUALITY CONTROL AND THE MEDICAL BOARD

Two of the most sensitive issues facing every hospital governing board, administration, and medical staff are quality control and medical staff discipline. I found that two formally organized bodies within the hospital structure—the joint conference committee, and the appointed medical board—provided an informed, authoritative, and equitable approach to handling these issues.

The Joint Conference Committee

One of the most valuable contributions to improved patient care (though I did not appreciate it until I came to New Haven) was the medical committee of the board of directors, which, together with representatives of the medical board and the administration, functioned as the joint conference committee. In discussions of problems of discipline or medical staff relationships, lay board members often put steel in the spines of the medical representatives, as one medical staff leader aptly put it. Nonmedical board members could not pass judgment on problems related to the specialized practice of medicine, but they were just as competent as anyone else to judge the integrity, responsibility, and character of a physician. They supplied a dispassionate point of view which helped clarify the thinking of physicians who were put in the position of having to judge or discipline friends and colleagues.

The Medical Board

The other body at the heart of the hospital's medical staff and patient-care program was the medical board. In hospitals large enough to have defined specialties, it once seemed to me appropriate to have as a nucleus for the medical board the chiefs of medicine, surgery, obstetrics-gynecology, pediatrics, radiology, pathology, and anesthesiology, as well as a chief of staff and the CEO of the hospital, whether or not he or she is a doctor. Now I would also include the person responsible for nursing as well as the chief of the family or general practice department, if the hospital were so organized. In some hospitals, chiefs of certain medical or surgical subspecialties are included—usually dependent upon the stature of the physician or the number of patients the service admits.

The hospital board encouraged the medical staff to organize and elect their own officers, and their president and past president were also on the medical board. The executive director of the hospital and the dean of the medical school were also full members. As we further developed our organizational and personal relationships, a hospital chief of staff was appointed by the board of directors. This officer was eventually accepted as the chairman of the medical board. Before this arrangement came into being, I had been serving as the chairman of the medical board, but I considered it more appropriate that as CEO I should be a member only.

The voting record of the hospital medical board demonstrates our working relationship. During my twenty-two years of membership on the board, only two decisions were made on a mixed vote. The members felt that if some opposed a decision—even if a substantial majority favored it—there might be something wrong. So the decision was usually postponed until the proposal could be further explored or modified.

One split vote that was allowed to become part of the record occurred after Paul Beeson, chairman of the Department of Medicine, moved to recommend to the board of directors that cigarettes not be sold in the hospital. This was soon after the American Cancer Society's first statistical studies on the link between cigarettes and cancer. To everyone's surprise, the motion carried by about 14 to 7. After a long silence, it was agreed that the recommendation be sent on through the joint conference committee to the board. Here again it was received with surprise—but after a couple of months Grace-New Haven became one of the first hospitals in the country to ban the sale of cigarettes on its premises.

DISCIPLINING THE MEDICAL STAFF

The medical board and the chiefs of service are obviously the principal officers to evaluate the quality of care and to discipline members of the staff when necessary. Unsatisfactory performance is usually first noted by the chief and his or her colleagues. As a rule, the chief discusses the deficiency with the offending physician and it is corrected. For example, at Grace-New Haven, the tissue committee once reported that an unusually high percentage of normal appendixes were being removed by a prominent community surgeon on the staff. The chief of surgery discussed the situation with the physician and the incidence of such surgery dropped. That was that! Another time, a prominent, elderly physician asked to see me about an idea he had. I listened to him for half an hour. After he left, I told his chief that I had not understood a word he had said and asked if anyone suspected that he was losing his grasp on reality. The reluctant answer was yes. This conversation resulted in a plan to induce the physician to retire. In the meantime, we arranged to have his colleagues and the resident staff monitor him and his hospital patients. Significantly, although the physician's colleagues were aware of his deterioration, the stimulus for corrective action had to come from the hospital administrator.

These examples delineate how the medical board, the chiefs of service, and the administration can work together informally to correct the medical staff. I do not wish to write a chapter on medical horror stories, but in order to underscore the importance of handling misbehavior quickly and fairly, I note here some distressing episodes that had to be handled by me and the medical board, sometimes with involvement of the hospital board.

Some of the unfortunate situations imprinted on my memory are cases of:

- A tenured professor and departmental chairman, liked by all, who was a chronic alcoholic and clearly deteriorating.
- A senior physician and department chairman with epilepsy, who was taking an increasing amount of tranquilizers and was obviously not alert much of the time.
- A psychiatrist who notified no one that one of his patients, a nurse with a morphine addiction, was stealing morphine from the patient division and substituting similar-looking tablets of a different drug.
- A physician who repeatedly ruptured the uterus when performing approved therapeutic abortions.
- A physician who insisted on prescribing naturopathic remedies for his cancer patients.
- A surgeon under psychiatric care who would appear at the nurses' station at two o'clock in the morning giving bizarre orders.
- A young physician who peformed an abortion on his girlfriend, a nurse.
- A doctor who kept referring patients to the hospital for bleeding hemorrhoids: many of them later proved to have cancers of the rectum—unnoticed because the doctor had made no rectal examinations.
- A surgeon whose long-standing alcoholism was being covered by his friends—even when he appeared drunk in the operating room.

The story of the alcoholic surgeon is a case study in how the hospital board and medical staff organization can save a brilliant physician from self-destruction. I was first introduced to the situation when the wife of a close friend was admitted in the middle of the night with a serious head injury. I called back an hour later and was told that she was in the operating room waiting for the surgeon. A half hour later, he had still not shown up, and other members of the surgical staff were taking care of her.

The next day I asked the reason for the delay in the operating room. It was like pulling teeth to get an answer, but finally it came out—the doctor had been too drunk to come in. I discussed this with the chief of surgery and learned to my amazement that the situation had been going on for years, and the surgeon's colleagues had been covering for him. He was a friend of mine. I told him of what I had heard and pointed out the obvious problems he and the hospital would face if his behavior continued. He assured me that he had recognized the problem and that it would not recur. I accepted this, but I told the chief of surgery, the director of nurses, and the operating room supervisor of my concern. Two weeks later, he appeared in the operating room drunk, and the resident staff and other surgeons had to take over the case.

What followed was one of the most unpleasant experiences of my career. The chief of surgery, the president of the hospital board, and I met with the surgeon. I reviewed his history, reminded him of the episode just two weeks earlier, and we presented two alternatives. The medical staff bylaws detailed the typical, complicated procedure through which a member of the medical staff could be disciplined or have hospital privileges reduced or withdrawn. We assured him that every detail would be followed if he so desired. Obviously, everyone in the hospital would eventually learn of the situation. He also had the option of immediately resigning his hospital privileges and consulting with a psychiatrist of his choice. No hospital privileges would be restored until the psychiatrist and the hospital agreed.

The surgeon finally chose the latter course. I told the psychiatrist of our interest in having him return to the staff. A month later he reported that the surgeon would probably always be an alcoholic; but his life was centered on surgery and his competence, when sober, was unsurpassed. The psychiatrist felt that our firm stand had made a profound impact on the surgeon, and that it would be appropriate and therapeutic for him to resume practice. He recommended that he continue to monitor the doctor; that the nursing, resident, and attending staff give clear warning if he came in drunk; and he said that the surgeon would allow his colleagues to take over if he ever started on a drinking spree.

Cynical practitioners in alcoholism treatment may laugh at the suggested solution. The board president, the chief of surgery, and I did not. The surgeon came back the following day and, until his death from unrelated causes a number of years later, he carried out his responsibilities most satisfactorily. He never talked to me again—I must have personified the hospital policeman for him—but I believe that the hospital, as represented by the chief of services, the board president, and the administrator, through our collective authority directed toward a high standard of patient care, preserved and prolonged the life and work of a brilliant physician.

The instances that I have listed are extremes. There were also many, many instances in which patient treatment was a matter of judgment, training, or philosophy. Every physician has seen his or her treatments turn out badly, and many of the best with whom I have reviewed the unfortunate outcome of a colleague's treatment have said, "There, but for the grace of God, go I." Thus, even the most conscientious physician will bend over backwards to avoid being critical of his associates, because the practice of medicine is not an exact science. This is another compelling reason for the members of the medical board and the medical chiefs to be independent of their colleagues—appointed by the hospital board and not elected by their associates.

HOSPITAL MECHANISMS FOR QUALITY CONTROL

Two mechanisms proved extremely helpful to the joint conference committee and the medical board in controlling the quality of professional care. The first was regular checking on the patients' progress. The second lay in the hospital privileges granted by the hospital board to the individual physician.

Monitoring Patient Care

This is one of the major contributions of the hospital standardization program established in 1917 by the American College of Surgeons. The program was reorganized in 1952 at the request of the college into the Joint Commission on the Accreditation of Hospitals (JCAH), with a representative governing board comprised of appointees from the AMA, the AHA, the American College of Physicians, the American College of Surgeons, and the Canadian Medical Association (which withdrew in 1959 to start its own program).

In the hospital, many instances of possible professional misconduct—infections following surgery, complications or deaths from anesthesia, abnormal drug reactions, unnecessary appendectomies or hysterectomies, and differences between diagnosis and the actual condition found during operation or at autopsy—could be detected relatively easily and checked against norms or expectations. When abnormalities occurred, the judgment or the competence of the doctor could be questioned. The sensitivity and the recollections of the chiefs of service, their colleagues, the resident staff, the nurses, the CEO, and the medical records staff all played informal roles in the monitoring of professional and hospital activities.

One case, already mentioned, involved a physician who ruptured a uterus during an attempted therapeutic abortion. This was not usual or accepted, but it *could* happen even with the best of gynecologists. However, it was unusual enough that its cause was questioned. To our collective embarrassment, a review of the doctor's records disclosed that over the past few years there had been at least two similar experiences—in one, an x-ray showed a small fetal thigh bone remaining in the woman's abdomen. The physician's surgical privileges were withdrawn and the chiefs of service and the various review committees became more careful to check abnormalities against doctors' records.

Hospital Privileges

The problems of assuring proper professional care for patients through the granting of privileges were clearly illustrated in a neighboring town whose hospital had about twenty-one doctors on its attending staff. Over two-thirds had surgical privileges, although all were formally listed as general practitioners and had no special surgical training. Specialists from New Haven on the consulting staff handled particularly complicated cases. The medical staff of this hospital engaged in a rather shady consultation practice. Every patient who was operated on there had a "consultation" in which the operating general practitioner had an associate enter a consultation note on the patient's chart. He would reciprocate later by "consulting" on a patient of his colleague.

The hospital board was made up of prominent individuals of the community, and by 1946 they had become dissatisfied with the quality of the medical care in the institution. A general practitioner in another community arranged for me to meet with members of the board. I told them that I thought their institution was a disgrace and asked them where they and their families went for care. Most said New Haven.

It took them a number of years to act, in part because the medical staff bylaws had been written years ago and were difficult to change. Finally, however, the board commissioned a prominent New Haven surgeon, who was on the consulting staff of the hospital, to prepare a new set of bylaws. He met with me to go over the draft, which spelled out surgical privileges, training, and competence. As we were reviewing the wording, he received an emergency telephone call. A patient in that hospital was being operated upon by a local general practitioner for what should have been a simple abdominal procedure. The doctor had found conditions that he either did not recognize or could not handle. The surgeon left my office in a hurry to drive to the hospital and take over the operation. Fortunately, the patient recovered.

This was the last straw. New bylaws were adopted, New Haven specialists were appointed as chiefs of service, and the surgical privileges of the twenty-one medical staff members were drastically reduced. Unfortunately, one doctor sued to retain his surgical privileges. As might be expected, a number of grateful and loyal patients were produced to testify to their faith in him. I had tried to stay in the background, but, to the administration's embarrassment as well as my own, our national colleagues in the AHA and the American College of Surgeons, who had encouraged the hospital administrator and the board to limit privileges, found that it might not be appropriate for them to testify. I thus became the expert witness, and I also invited Nathaniel Faxon, who had recently retired as general director of the Massachusetts General Hospital, to support the hospital's position. The hospital won the suit, which became a landmark decision on staff privileges and the responsibilities of hospitals in Connecticut.

Although this experience was a glaring example of how untrained physicians could improperly use hospital facilities, it also underscored the fact that a properly organized and managed hospital can ensure good professional care. I had not up to then been aware that the granting of privileges was a problem for hospital governing boards and their corporate institutions. It had been relatively simple at Strong Memorial Hospital in Rochester—all physicians on the hospital staff had faculty appointments in the school of medicine, as was the case in most university teaching hospitals. But in New Haven I learned how complicated the problem of hospital privileges became in a smaller community with only two hospitals. It was not a simple matter of granting hospital privileges to specialists only, nor could one be overly selective and depend upon the other hospital in town to give privileges to all other physicians. Of course, if there is only one hospital in a community or a region, the problem is intensified. A number of principles evolved in New Haven that seemed fair for the practitioners and the patients. Probably the two most important factors were (1) the power or authority that could be exerted by the hospital through the granting of privileges; and (2) the hospital's responsibility to consider the welfare of the patient and the quality of care that he or she would receive from those given privileges.

General practitioners are an excellent example. At Grace-New Haven, general practitioners had medical privileges and were under the supervision of the chief of the medical community service. If approved by the chiefs of obstetrics-gynecology and pediatrics, they were also given privileges for normal obstetrics and infant care. This worked for years to the satisfaction of the general practitioners, the obstetric- gynecology and pediatric staff, and the patients. But, with the exception of the general practitioners, limited privileges were not granted. It was difficult enough to screen physicians applying for the usual privileges without having to certify to the board that a doctor was competent to perform an appendectomy, but not to remove a gallbladder, and so on. We felt that, if a surgeon were allowed to open an abdomen to take out an appendix, he or she should be prepared to handle whatever other complications were found. Undoubtedly there are cases in which these arbitrary restrictions are unduly limiting, and they also may not be practical in all hospitals. An important part of any solution, therefore, is to recognize the fallibility of even the best physician and to set up checks and reviews that will enable the medical staff, the CEO, and the board to ascertain that the care rendered is as safe and as comprehensive as needed.

As the physician-population ratio in a community grows, the board may have to restrict the number of professionals to whom they grant privileges. This requires difficult policy decisions. We started facing this problem in New Haven in the 1960s, but we never advanced beyond the belief that it was safer for the community if the hospital granted physicians limited admitting privileges rather than excluding them from the hospital. We examined the number of specialized procedures that a physician might expect to carry out during a year, and, if these were expected to fall below an established minimum, such privileges were not granted. Gynecological operations were gradually restricted to those with specific credentials and demonstrated experience.

One way to limit privileges is through the custom whereby only specialists practice in the hospital, and the family physician or general practitioner cares for the patients before and after their hospital stay. This was the policy in the Hunterdon Medical Center in New Jersey, and it is the rule in Great Britain. It is a pattern worth exploring, but it is more important to make sure that the physician responsible for the continuing care of the patient is not excluded from contact with the patient when he or she is in the hospital under specialized care. This was our attitude.

The problem of responsibility confronting the hospital board was complicated in the spring of 1983 by the proposal to the JCAH that its standards refer to a "professional staff" for a hospital staff rather than the traditional "medical staff." This was intended to recognize the growing number of nonphysician health care practitioners in hospitals. It is difficult to separate the board's concern for the most equitable means of assuring the best care for patients, on the one hand, from tradition and custom and doctors' suspicions of allied health professionals, on the other. The contribution of these health professionals and the need for lower health-care costs must enter into the final policy decisions.

In New Haven in 1946, there were already many nonphysician professionals caring for patients. Dentists had hospital privileges—the hospital bylaws actually referred to the "medical and dental staff." There were also podiatrists, psychologists, social workers, physiotherapists, speech therapists, hearing specialists, and other professionals working in the hospital. The issue of hospital privileges, to the board and the medical staff leaders at Grace-New Haven, was this: people given privileges in the hospital must render adequate professional care to the hospital patients. Whether they were defined as medical, dental, or professional was immaterial. The hospital was responsible for total care of patients and that responsibility extended to those to whom it afforded privileges.

We had no trouble with dentists. They had special training and skills that physicians did not have. We did require that, if a dental patient were hospitalized, he or she be treated like any other patient. His or her condition was considered as a whole, involving a physician as well as a dentist. This policy also applied to other specialized health professionals to whom the hospital granted privileges. Although some hospitals— from legal pressure or custom—have allowed nonmedical health professionals to care for patients in the hospital without medical supervision, we merely assumed that any patient entering the hospital was our responsibility as well as that of the admitting professional, so we expected the care provided to be comprehensive.

The increasing number of nonphysician health professionals and the narrowing scope of the medical specialist may lead to problems in patient care. This is why the family physician should follow up on a patient who is being operated on by a specialist, and why medical supervision of patients who are sick enough to be hospitalized by a dentist or other health professional is necessary.

THE PHYSICIAN AND ORGANIZED MEDICINE

I have found it difficult over the years to understand the shift in the thought processes of physicians as individuals, on the one hand, and as representatives of a medical organization, on the other. I found this shifting viewpoint in members of the medical staff; and as I began to broaden my connections with county, state, and national organizations, as well as with the specialty societies, the same dichotomy appeared. I almost always worked amicably and constructively with physicians as individuals or in committees, but there always loomed a barrier to over-come—the "party line." When the laboriously developed policies or agreements were finally presented to the organization, they were often drastically modified following relatively short deliberation, summarily rejected, or later reversed. This may have been partly our fault for present-ing unsatisfactory recommendations, but part of the explanation, I believe, is that organized medicine is more conservative than many of its individual members. Economics also seem to be far more important than is admitted.

I have never privately practiced medicine, but I recognize the com-plications that physicians face in practice today. Public relations, govern-ment, the threat of litigation, fixed fee schedules, unions, medical and health-care corporations, and those mysterious forces of the marketplace and competition interfere with their practice and their enjoyment of their profession. Another problem doctors face is the tremendous increase in the amount of knowledge required and the resultant pressure to become more and more specialized, with narrowing gun-barrel vision. It is now more difficult to spend time talking to patients and learning of their questions and fears. Reimbursement schedules are not very generous for this type of office visit—procedures, tests, and special examinations provide more income for the same amount of time.[3]

Another problem is the increasing number of physicians. There is now a surplus of physicians in the country, or at least a marked imbalance in distribution, just as there is a surplus of hospital beds. The fault lies as much with the government as with the health care industry. For many years, Stanford, Rochester, and Yale, for example, all admitted compara-bly small numbers of students into their medical schools and were quite satisfied with the results. But the federal government offered political and financial inducements to all medical schools to increase their enrollments and encouraged universities to start new medical schools. Now that the production of physicians has increased remarkably, pressure—primarily withdrawal of educational and research subsidies—is now being placed on medical schools to lower enrollment. Medical schools now must seek

3. Benson Roe summarizes this problem well in his comments on remuneration for procedural services as contrasted to cognitive services. *New England Journal of Medicine* 313, 20 (November, 1985): 1286–89.

more income from clinical practice and patient fees. The major academic health centers will soon be facing even more serious problems in the financing of graduate medical education and in caring for the medically indigent.

An advantage to the surplus will be that hiring of graduates of foreign medical schools will be reconsidered. Although some of these graduates are excellent physicians, many do not meet minimal standards of competence. I have often wondered how medical staffs and administration of some hospitals rationalize the employment of these graduates on their resident staffs. Both staff and patient frequently have difficulty communicating with these doctors, and sometimes there are frank reservations regarding their training and competence.

ORGANIZED MEDICINE, THE STATE, AND QUALITY CONTROL

My primary problem with organized medicine is its reluctance to monitor or control the professional activities of its members. An impressive record has been developed over the years in opposing charlatans, quacks, and useless or harmful medication—but not in disciplining the small percentage of inadequate or incompetent physicians. I used to talk to Creighton Barker, for years the secretary of the Connecticut State Board of Medical Examiners, about poor medical practice in the community. He pointed out the limits of the state board's powers. Under its regulations, a fault had to be truly egregious before it could act. The board usually had to wait for a specific complaint from the patient, the family, or another physician. Moreover, the disciplinary actions open to the board were severe, usually involving rescinding the doctor's license. Dr. Barker also frankly discussed the attitude of organized medicine at the county and state level toward the quality of medicine practiced by their members. Members of these organizations were extremely hesitant to judge their peers. I was disturbed by this, for it was taken for granted that this was a primary concern and responsibility of those same physicians as members of the hospital staff.

I best expressed my attitude in February, 1954, when Walter Martin, soon to be president of the AMA, and I spoke on hospital-physician relations to the state meeting of the Medical Society of the County of New York.[4] I discussed the authority in reviewing, evaluating, controlling, and disciplining the professional actions of their colleagues. I pointed out the ease of constructive action on the part of the organized hospital staff, as

4. A. Snoke, "Hospital-Physician Relationships—The Hospital View," *New York Medicine* 10, 6 (March 20, 1954), 220.

contrasted to their authority as individual practitioners, and as compared to the type of authority possible for a county medical society. I noted that, although I had been trained only in medicine and pediatrics, my medical licenses in California, New York, and Connecticut were very permissive. As far as the state was concerned, I could perform neurosurgery if my conscience permitted and a patient were dumb enough to let me. (However, any reputable hospital would have refused to give me such privileges because I was not competent.)

These comments still seem appropriate thirty years later, even with the substantial changes that have resulted from the removal of charitable immunity for eleemosynary institutions and the great increase in medical malpractice suits. They may also provide a partial answer to the criticism of David Axelrod, commissioner of health in New York state, of the failure of organized medicine to control its own members.[5] He said that the problem of physician misconduct in New York was overwhelming, and hundreds of complaints had piled up because the state was unable to handle the load. But many of the examples cited—illegal prescriptions of methaqualone, Medicaid fraud, misuse of x-rays, and the practice of needlessly "ping-ponging" patients from one specialist to another to generate fees—were most frequently associated with ambulatory care and not susceptible to control by organized medicine—particularly if the doctor was not a member of the medical society.

In this case, much as I love to needle my associates in organized medicine, I question whether they are guilty of anything except not officially recognizing and pressing for a solution to the problem. A hospital can take away a physician's privileges, and a medical society can censure or expel a member. The state licensing board, however, has—or can be given—the authority to restrict or remove the physician's license to practice. States and/or federated boards must also work together so that miscreants do not just move their offices across the state line and continue to practice as before, now not an unusual occurrence. It should be the joint responsibility of organized medicine, state health officials, and state legislatures to develop a more comprehensive approach to controlling the quality of health care in the community, such as has been practiced for many years within the voluntary hospital. I don't have the slightest doubt that state boards of health and state medical examining boards can attract conscientious, competent, courageous, and respected physicians to function in such capacities. I had them as chiefs of service in the hospitals with which I was associated, and most of the leaders of organized medicine

5. Published in the *New York Times*, April 13, 1983.

with whom I have worked could assume this authority. I also suggest that lay individuals of the caliber that I encountered on hospital boards and in the CHA be included on any review and disciplinary board.

Finally, I wish that my colleagues in the medical profession were more aware of the erosion of the public's trust in physicians. From a healer, the image of the physician has dwindled to that of a wheeler-dealer. (It is perhaps appropriate here to repeat a wisecrack made by John A. D. Cooper, recently retired as president of the Association of American Medical Colleges: "I hope you recognize that with the present efforts to mercantilize medicine, physicians are not scholarly professionals, who care for patients. They are entrepreneurs, who market their products to consumers, who purchase them." I suspect he classifies hospital administrators somewhat similarly.) I know my colleagues' concern for the welfare of their patients, and I also know that many of them are willing to help in extraordinary times and places. I am also impressed with people's respect for their personal doctors. But the new physician unions, the doctors' parking lots full of Cadillacs, Lincoln-Continentals, and Mercedes, and the expensive homes owned by physicians in exclusive sections of the community are not helpful illustrations of what I think it means to be part of this most satisfying profession.

It is not easy for the physician of today to see the patient as a whole. The amount of knowledge he or she has to absorb merely to keep up to date is already enormous and rapidly expanding. Medical schools face the same problem as they try to prepare young doctors to care for people in this environment. In 1979, Dean Robert Berliner delivered the following comments to the Yale Corporation:

> We believe we are educating people to give the best possible medical care. I maintain that doctors do not deliver health care, but rather medical care, and although the two are related, they are very different things. Medical care is the interaction between the physician and his or her patient. There are many features of our social structure and behavior that are detrimental to health—features that physicians individually and collectively have neither the competence nor the power to modify significantly. Those preventative measures that physicians as individuals can and should offer constitute an important, but, unfortunately, not a very large category. The major role of the physician is still the care of sick people— one at a time.

This is probably the overriding philosophy of health care among academic research–oriented administrators. Others who are high in medical academic circles may take a broader view of patient care, but opinion seems sharply divided between those who favor emphasis on research and the "publish or perish" philosophy, on the one hand; and those who prefer a

balanced "three-legged stool," considering people care as equally important, on the other.

I believe these attitudes can be combined. I look back at my personal
experience over fifty years with many physicians in academia, in hospital
and community practice, and in isolated, rural areas. The attitude of these
colleagues of mine can be summed up in the words of one of my best
friends, David Rytand. He has received many awards from Stanford
University, but he recently described his two greatest achievements as
these: "I taught students, and I listened to patients."

MALPRACTICE

Malpractice has now become a very serious problem that is not only
increasing the cost of health care substantially but is also affecting noticea-
bly the practice of medicine. For many years, malpractice was a relatively
minor problem to physicians and an even smaller one to hospitals.
Charitable immunity for the eleemosynary institutions was taken for
granted. The hospital was a nonprofit institution, and it did not seem
appropriate, nor was it legal under the trust fund doctrine, to penalize it
financially for mistakes. The attitude toward physicians' conduct was not
much more punitive, nor were legal actions or settlements a particular
problem, as evidenced by the relatively low malpractice insurance premiums through the 1950s. I was not particularly disturbed as state after
state removed the charitable immunity of nonprofit hospitals, for I was
aware of accidents and inadequacies, and I believed that, not only did
patients deserve reimbursement for improper care, but penalties encouraged more careful monitoring of performance.

I became more aware of the problems of malpractice when I came to
New Haven. Although charitable immunity still existed in Connecticut in
1946, I developed the practice of reviewing possible cases of improper care
with the attending physician. Together we decided how to adjust the
hospital bill and the professional fee, and how to correct the patient's
problem. Usually we canceled all charges and readmitted the patient for
whatever remedial procedures were necessary, with no additional
charge.

Within a few years, we took out malpractice insurance for the hospital
and its salaried physicians (radiologists, anesthesiologists, pathologists,
physiatrists, and so on), and Yale took out insurance for the other salaried
medical school faculty. To educate myself, I became the messenger for the
record room when a patient's records were subpoenaed in a malpractice
suit. After one or two suits involving members of the resident staff, I

arranged to have the insurance company's lawyers represent these residents, and later I arranged to have our entire resident staff covered. At the time, the additional premium for covering the entire resident staff was negligible. A few years later, a staff nurse was involved in a malpractice suit, so we arranged to have the nurses covered—again, for a negligible increase. Strong Memorial and Grace-New Haven hospitals were early leaders in arranging such coverage, but within a few years the entire "poison ivy" league of teaching hospitals (see chapter 6) covered all staff as a matter of course.

For a number of years all malpractice cases were handled on a part-time basis by an administrative associate who also handled public relations, the women's auxiliary, and community relations. I continued as the record room messenger so I could learn about court procedures and the attitudes and knowledge of the judges and lawyers in these cases. As the years went on, I was often asked to function as an expert witness for either patient or hospital in malpractice suits. I always reviewed the complete story or record before deciding whether to participate. I learned both when I participated and when I did not, and I came to the reluctant conclusion that at times doctors and hospitals were careless, so that patients deserved compensation, and that lawyers were necessary even though they sometimes seemed more interested in their fees than in the merits of the case.

A prestigious legal firm in Texas once asked me to appear at a case in which a doctor and a hospital were being sued because of the death of a baby at birth. The doctor was obviously at fault, but they wanted me to help defend the hospital. After reviewing all the records and depositions, my wife and I told the hospital attorneys that the records showed the physician had no formal residency training in obstetrics, had been given complete obstetric privileges in the hospital for six years or more, during which he had handled fewer than five deliveries a year; he had never handled an abnormal delivery, nor had he any training in abnormal obstetrics. In this case, he had foreseen a possible breech delivery several days earlier, but he had not come to the hospital until several hours after being notified of the woman's admission in labor. When he arrived, birth had already begun, and the baby had to be removed piecemeal. There was no question that the doctor should be punished, but I also thought it outrageous that he had been given unlimited obstetrical privileges. I said that I would be a ticking time bomb if I appeared for the hospital, because I would testify that they had been wrong in granting such privileges to this physician. The lawyers said at first that these privileges were customary in the area. I said that I knew many of the hospital administrators in that city and doubted it. If they disagreed, they should get a local expert to support their position. The end result was (1) they agreed that I would be a ticking time bomb; and (2) they settled the case out of court.

There are legitimate cases of malpractice. When the hospital, the physician, or both can be shown to be at fault, the patient should be compensated for the costs incurred and for the damage. The problem is always deciding what is a reasonable amount. There are also situations in which unfortunate results occur regardless of the competence of the physician or the hospital. I have investigated many such abnormal occurrences with my medical and hospital staffs and have encountered situations in which we could find neither any appropriate explanation nor any evidence of negligence. These were occurrences in which neither the medical nor the hospital staff needed to be defensive or evasive. After careful review, our only conclusion was that an inexplicable complication had occurred for which we could not fix any blame. Cases such as these are the reason I challenge the present system in which malpractice decisions are made by juries. Members of the jury often do not have the knowledge they need to decide wisely. To make matters worse, they must make judgments on the basis of the diametrically opposed opinions of so-called medical experts and lawyers on both sides of the controversy. I question the ability of a lay jury to make an informed and fair decision in this highly specialized situation.

It is not only the large judgments awarded to the patients or their families but also the substantial contingency fees and the steadily mounting cost of malpractice insurance to hospitals and physicians that are troublesome. The impact of malpractice suits upon health care costs is now assuming greater importance. This cost is borne eventually by the patient, either directly or through third party payments and insurance. Hospital costs prove the point. As I mentioned, malpractice premiums were negligible in the 1950s and 1960s. In 1970, Yale-New Haven's annual malpractice premiums had mounted to about $150,000. In 1971, the premium doubled. By 1985, it is estimated that commercial insurance would have cost the hospital over $10 million per year, during which time the hospital assigned five full-time staff members, significant administrative support, and a part-time medical consultant to what is now termed "risk management." Because of the hospital's record and performance, it has been able to participate in an alternative insurance program that has saved approximately $10 million over six years. But premiums are expected again to more than double during the next year or so, and two additional full-time staff may be needed, bringing the risk management staff budget alone to approximately $150,000 annually.

Premium increases for individual physicians are just as startling. Annual malpractice premiums once cost only a few hundred dollars a year, but now they range from $5,000 to $100,000 dollars, dependent upon the specialty and the location of the physician's practice. Many competent, conscientious physicians are retiring early from practice, because their premiums, along with the cost of maintaining an office, require an expenditure of time and effort that is neither enjoyable nor rewarding. Abandonment of obstetric practice is now a significant phenomenon in Connecticut. A survey by the Connecticut State Medical Society in 1985 revealed that up to 20 percent of the obstetricians in Connecticut had either abandoned or limited their practice, and others were refusing high-risk cases. Malpractice insurance appeared to be the primary reason—costing many of these physicians over $50,000 a year. Cesarean sections are also on the increase as a result of the need to practice defensive medicine. This obviously increases the cost to the patient.

An additional factor that is virtually impossible to measure is the cost of defensive medicine—laying careful foundations for successful defense against malpractice claims. Additional examinations and procedures are now carried out routinely because of the possibility of being held negligent if they are not done. How easy for the prosecuting lawyer and his or her expert witness to damn the doctor or the hospital if some procedure—no matter how esoteric—was not done.

As the direct and indirect costs of malpractice continue to mount, demand is growing for limitation on awards and attorney's fees or percentages, and for various types of no-fault, deductibles, and co-insurance. Whether these are implemented will depend largely upon legislation at the state and federal levels, and it is not difficult to anticipate the objections of the trial lawyers. I can also foresee legislators' hesitance to change the present system when so many of them are lawyers. I expect that lawyers and their organizations are no less interested in their pocketbooks than are their medical counterparts. But the escalating cost of health care may well demand critical review of the system of evaluation, judgment, and awards. I doubt whether the growing problem of malpractice can ever be solved merely by tinkering with our existing system. Instead, consideration should be given to an entirely different approach.

Medical care and hospital procedures are just as complicated as bankruptcy law, SEC actions, tax court, maritime law, public utility hearings, liquor control and trade commissions, worker's compensation, National Labor Relations Board activities, and a score of other legal questions in which lay individuals are not expected to have the expertise to make sophisticated decisions. What is needed is an expert referee, judge, or select panel that could evaluate the merits of each case. Again, I believe that individuals can be found who would function intelligently and equitably in such a position. In the hospital, it did not take me long to learn which physicians, nurses, or other health care professionals I could trust to think objectively. It may be blasphemy to question the system of judgment by a jury of peers. But when I learned that other complicated legal or judicial matters have been accepted as inappropriate for a lay jury, I wondered whether the jury system was the best for this situation. Do opposing lawyers fighting for a percentage of the judgment represent a sensible system for resolving a serious medical and social problem? Mounting costs, direct and indirect effects on the type of care rendered, and the possibility of many other inequities warrant a substantial critical review of the system.

The phenomena of increasing awards and premiums has now extended through society at large. Astronomic liability awards, the plethora of lawyers encouraging suits and then pocketing a huge percentage of the awards, and the inability of many municipalities, companies, and organizations to afford liability insurance are becoming disturbing facts of life. We must not merely duck the issue by assuming that insurance will pay for the awards and that lawyers are money-hungry. There are legitimate malpractice actions, but health providers and the government must do a better job in enforcing quality controls for all health care. Now that tort reform is an issue in most states, the medical profession, which may well have stimulated this explosion, may benefit. Yet, regardless of what legislation might result, physicians and hospitals still have the responsibility to discipline and control themselves.

5

The Salaried Physician

In 1930–31, when I was a student at the Stanford Medical School, we were told that the professor of radiology, Edward Chamberlain, had resigned because he was dissatisfied with the way he was paid by the hospital and the medical school. Apparently he received a salary. This meant little to us other than regret at losing a stimulating clinical teacher. Fortunately, his successor, Robert Newell, was his equal in teaching, diagnostic acumen, and attention to house staff and students. He seemed to be quite satisfied with his salaried arrangement. Not until years later, when I became involved with the AMA and the national organizations of hospital-based specialists, did I discover that salary was the subject of a never-ending dialogue. It still is.

The primary problem areas in the 1930s were the hospital-based specialties—radiology, pathology, and anesthesiology. But the issue soon extended to include electrocardiology, electroencephalography, physiatry, rehabilitation medicine, inhalation therapy, psychiatry, emergency services, and, later on, a myriad of subspecialties that usually developed first in hospitals. Debates and negotiations never really faced the issue squarely. I readily understood and supported the several alternatives advocated by the specialty societies and medical organizations: fee-for-service charges, a percentage of the net or gross departmental income, even the leasing of specific hospital facilities to a physician or a group that charged patients directly. But I never understood why the professional organizations so adamantly opposed the concept of physicians receiving a salary from either the hospital or the medical school. Many of the specialists believed, theoretically at least, that their responsibilities to patients might be more difficult to carry out by loss of independence. Some were suspicious of administrators. Some may have felt that their

57

colleagues would consider them second-class doctors if they did not bill patients independently. Nevertheless, their continued uncompromising opposition persuaded me that their pocketbooks were also a major source of concern.

This rather irreverent attitude was affected by an early experience in Rochester. Strong Memorial hospital had always used nurse anesthetists, but by the early 1940s serious thought was being given to bringing in physician anesthesiologists. Since other full-time chiefs of service were salaried, the university and the hospital planned to set up a department with salaried physicians. A highly regarded anesthesiologist came to see Dr. MacLean to declare that he and his fellows were strongly opposed to this arrangement. Dr. MacLean later called me in to tell me of the conversation. I could not understand why he kept interrupting himself with laughter. Finally it came out: after the anesthesiologist had delivered a long monologue on the evils of salary, Dr. MacLean explained why he felt that a salaried medical anesthesiologist was needed in the institution and mentioned that it had been suggested that his visitor might be interested in this salaried position. The response was a thoughtful question as to what the salary range might be. Another early flareup of the salary issue occurred while I was in Rochester. In 1944, the Rochester Hospital Service Corporation (Blue Cross) was considering a new contract for its subscribers that would cover all hospital services. The County Medical Society objected to the inclusion of x-rays in the contract. In my first attempt to break into print on the subject, I argued that the inclusion of x-rays did not mean any change in the professional status of the radiologist: clinical pathology, for example, had long been included in hospital service contracts, yet the pathologist was not adversely affected. Whether the radiologist was paid a salary, a commission, or a fee was immaterial if the quality of service was not impaired and if he or she and the hospital were satisfied. I further noted that x-rays were already included in hospital service contracts in forty-four Blue Cross plans. I don't recall whether the editorial was printed, but radiology did finally become part of the service contract.

As assistant director, I was responsible for dealing with the radiologists at SMH. Our personal relationships were good, and their status in the hospital was the same as that of all the other physicians. The community attending staff had no reservations about the professional competence of their specialist colleagues in radiology. Indeed, in my associations with hospitals and medical schools in Stanford, Rochester, and New Haven, I found that the salaried physicians were competent and concerned for their patients and the administrators did not interfere with their responsibilities. It was rare indeed for administrators to interfere with doctors' professional activities, whatever the financial arrangement.

My arrival in New Haven in 1946 coincided with an escalating hospital-physician confrontation that eventually exploded around 1950. It subsided somewhat by 1960, but occasional skirmishes have continued to break out to the present. I became involved in these battles in part because of my growing official relationship with the AHA. As mentioned, my attitudes were also influenced by my respect for salaried teachers and professional colleagues in the institutions with which I was associated. I felt strongly that many of the criticisms directed at salaried financial relationships with the medical school and hospital were specious, self-serving, and unfair. However, from 1946 on, ethics, economics, licensing, specialty boards, professional independence, personalities, sanctions, attorneys general, courts, hospitals, national health legislation, and social sanctions became inextricably entangled in the arguments and actions of the medical specialty organizations, state medical societies, and the AMA.

In 1939, the Principles of Relationship between Hospitals and Radiologists, Pathologists, and Anesthesiologists were adopted jointly by the AHA; the Radiological Inter-Society Committee, officially representing the American College of Radiology, American Roentgen Ray Society, and the Radiological Society of North America; a special committee representing the American Society of Clinical Pathologists.[1] The principles were again published in 1946, with the additional endorsement of the Council on Professional Practice of the AHA, which included a number of distinguished physicians; the Council on Medical Education and Hospitals of the AMA; and the American College of Surgeons. Included in the principles was the statement:

Inasmuch as no one basis of financial arrangement between a hospital and its radiologist [or other named specialty] would seem to be applicable or suitable in all instances, that basis should be followed which would best meet the local situation. This may be on the basis of salary, commission, or privileged rental, but in no instance should either the hospital or the radiologist [or other named specialty] exploit the other or the patient.

Attitudes changed rather rapidly. When the AHA reprinted the principles in 1951, footnotes indicated that approval had been withdrawn by the American College of Radiology on September 24, 1950, and by the American Society of Anesthesiologists on July 17, 1950. The executive director of the American Society of Pathologists wrote in 1959 that it had

1. AHA Council on Professional Practice, "Principles of Relationship Between Hospitals and Radiologists, Anesthesiologists, Pathologists," Annual Report, 1939

also withdrawn approval in a Statement of Principles Relating to the Practice of Pathology, December, 1958.

THE HESS COMMITTEE

The Hess Committee was appointed by the AMA in January, 1948, to study the various resolutions on hospital-physician relations passed by the AMA House of Delegates and to confer with other organizations. In January, 1949, the House of Delegates approved a report of the Hess Committee as revised by the Reference Committee. In December, 1949, the House rescinded its approval of the revised report (apparently on advice of legal counsel) and referred the original report back to the original committee. In June, 1950, the Hess Committee resubmitted its report, which was approved by the House of Delegates after amendment. Finally, in December, 1951, the House of Delegates approved "Guides for Conduct of Physicians in Relationships with Institutions," submitted by the AMA Board of Trustees to be substituted for all previous reports. The wait for these guidelines was frustrating, but the ways organizations and individuals selectively used those portions that seemed to justify their interests were even more so.

I came to know Elmer Hess as I became more active in the AHA and he became president of the AMA. During the Hess Committee turmoil, I had considered him a prejudiced ogre, so I was surprised and delighted to find him decent, fair, and level-headed. This was borne out by the history of the report, how it was originally presented, and how it was received and modified by the AMA House of Delegates. The report came to the board of trustees and the House of Delegates several times. Each time it reflected a far more reasonable, more realistic, and less dogmatic point of view than that of the document eventually accepted by the AMA.[2] Dr. Hess's attitude was well described by an article in *Modern Hospital*.[3] After the final recommendation of the House's reference committee was completed, Dr. Hess "suggested that his name should now be removed from the report, and the chairman of the reference committee indicated that this had already been done. 'Thank God,' sighed Dr. Hess, whose own views on the subject were considerably less militant than those expressed in the report which has carried his name. When the House of Delegates

2. "Guides for Conduct of Physicians in Relationship with Institutions," *jama* 147, 117 (December 22, 1951), 1684.

3. "AMA Approves Hess Report Substitute," *Modern Hospital* 78, 1 (January, 1952), 35–56, 140–144.

approved the new 'Guides' without further discussion, the Hess Report qua Hess Report became an unhappy memory."

Unfortunately the new guidelines did not settle anything. Instead, controversy erupted over their various possible interpretations—particularly this statement:

A physician should not dispose of his professional attainments or services to any hospital, corporation or lay body by whatsoever name called or however organized under terms or conditions which permit the sale of the services for a fee.

This sentence was understood to amend the Principles of Medical Ethics established by the AMA and interpreted by its Judicial Council when suspected infractions occurred. The new statement was considered applicable to salaried physicians employed by voluntary hospitals, such as full-time radiologists, anesthesiologists, and pathologists, as well as salaried medical school clinicians. Consequently, a salaried physician in a hospital was considered unethical if the hospital charged for his services. Failure to reconcile the "Guides" and the AMA Principles of Ethics caused misunderstandings. As a result, the ethics and legality of practicing medicine on salary became a new battleground.

ETHICS

The ethics of physicians and of the practice of medicine have long been a matter of great importance to the profession and the AMA has been involved intimately in the subject. It developed the Principles of Medical Ethics and created the Judicial Council to function as their final interpreter—essentially the Supreme Court on medical ethics. During the 1940s, the ethics of certain methods of remuneration became a popular subject for debate, and the AMA's 1951 "Guides" were seized upon by specialty groups and medical societies as proof positive that physicians on salary were unethical and subject to punishment. It is unfortunate that the subject of ethics can be diverted from poor professional practice or improper personal behavior to condemn any economic or social arrangement that individuals or organizations think is against their interests. The March, 1952 declaration of the American Society of Anesthesiologists that "it is unethical for a practicing physician anesthesiologist to enter into any relationship with a corporation which permits that corporation to offer his services for a fee" was solemnly quoted to every anesthesiologist who might be offered a salary.

By 1951, I became tired of hearing salaries and hospital or medical school billing for physician services termed unethical, and I decided to challenge the AMA directly. I wrote a letter for the signature of George Stevenson, the president of the board of Grace-New Haven. It was addressed to Edward R. Cunniffe, chairman of the Judicial Council of the AMA. I used as a basis for the hospital's concern the Connecticut State Medical Society's resolution of 1951 directed to the Judicial Council of the AMA. The society stated that the Yale School of Medicine employed physicians on salary whose professional fees were collected by the school of medicine's Clinical Practice Office. This practice, claimed the society, directly violated the AMA's principles of ethics and the recommendations of the Hess Committee. I confirmed that these physicians were on salary and that their fees were billed and collected by the medical school, and I added that this also applied to salaried radiologists, anesthesiologists, and physiatrists employed by the hospital. I pointed out that if these physicians were found to be unethical by the Judicial Council, it would be their duty to request that the AMA's Council on Medical Education and Hospitals remove our hospital from the approved lists for internships and residencies. This would imply that paying salaries to physicians was on par with failure to maintain proper filing systems for laboratory or clinical records or allowing inadequately trained personnel to care for patients. I then outlined the existing internships and residencies in the hospital, and pointed out that many distinguished physicians had come from this teaching and clinical environment. I challenged the AMA either to declare the salaried physician unethical and remove its approval of the intern and residence training at Grace-New Haven, or agree that physicians on salary in a medical school or hospital were not unethical.

The first letter was dated June 2, 1951. There was no answer. A second letter was then sent. Finally, in October, Dr. Cunniffe responded that the matter was under investigation. Again, nothing happened. In August, 1952, I wrote Dr. Cunniffe and the Judicial Council under my own signature and sent copies of the letters to everyone I could think of—particularly to the secretary and general manager of the AMA, George Lull, to the AHA, and to my counterparts in the other major teaching hospitals on the eastern seaboard.

The responses that I began to receive were fascinating. Edwin L. Crosby, then director at the Johns Hopkins Hospital, wrote that they were facing the same problem and were most intrigued by my letters. Had I by any chance employed the famous attorney Thurman Arnold to write my letter? I was flattered. Dean Clark of Massachusetts General Hospital wrote that he was initiating a parallel series of questions to the AMA. Dr. Lull then wrote me that neither MGH nor I had anything to worry about.

None of us in the major teaching hospitals ever believed that we had anything to worry about. But we were dissatisfied with the lack of formal action.

Finally, in September, 1952, I received a formal answer from the Judicial Council, which stated,

It is the opinion of the Judicial Council that it is neither the sense nor the intent of Section 6, Article VI, Chapter III of the Principles of Medical Ethics to establish as ethical or to proscribe as unethical any particular financial arrangement—any term or condition—by which a physician disposes of his professional attainment or services.

And eventually, Dr. Lull wrote to Dr. Clark, quoting from the AMA's Principles of Medical Ethics:

Chapter III, Article VI. Section 6. Title: Purveyal of Medical Service—A physician should not dispose of his professional attainments or services to any hospital, lay body, organization, group or individual, or whatsoever by whatever name called, or however organized, under terms or conditions which permit exploitation of the services of the physician for the financial profit of the agency concerned. Such a procedure is beneath the dignity of professional practice and is harmful alike to the profession of medicine and the welfare of the people.

Dr. Lull also enclosed an excerpt from the minutes of the Judicial Council meeting of November 25, 1952:

The chairman stated the opinion of the council that the Principles of Medical Ethics are not overruled by the general principles set forth in the "Hess Report" and that the "Hess Report" is advisory. The chairman also stated that the problem presented by Dr. Clark is similar to the one with which the Yale University physicians are concerned at Grace-New Haven Community Hospital.

The Judicial Council's September, 1952, statement was reaffirmed in 1958.[4] Nevertheless, the argument continued, involving medical societies, organizations, and the hospitals at local, regional, and national levels. In 1956, a proposal was made to the Federated State Medical Licensing Board that it recommend an addition to its "model" medical practice bill, providing the following grounds for suspension or revocation of license: "practicing medicine as a partner, agent or employee of a person who does not own a license to practice medicine, or practicing medicine as an employee of an association or corporation." This was to be added to already accepted unethical, antisocial, or unprofessional acts such as drug addiction, murder, rape, and so on. The proposal was defeated, but only after a number of people pointed out that many of

4. "Principles of Medical Ethics: Opinions and Reports of the Judicial Council," *jama* special ed. (June 7, 1958), 37.

those participating in the discussion, along with officers of the AMA and the state medical societies, and many of the respected leaders in medical schools and communities would become liable to lose their licenses under the proposal. Similar legislation in North Dakota was defeated a few years later, and this was the last gasp for legislated economic ethics.

The Hess reports of 1950 and 1951, the "Guides," and their various interpretations by medical organizations and individuals prompted the AMA and the AHA, in June, 1951, to set up a joint committee at the level of the board of trustees to review the situation. I sat on this committee, along with the president, the president-elect, the chairman of the board of trustees, and three other members of the board of the AMA; as well as the immediate past president, the president-elect, and members of the AHA board of trustees. It was one of the most stimulating and pleasant episodes of my career, and the first time in my experience that the national leaders of the hospitals and the medical profession sat around the table in a friendly give-and-take atmosphere to review common problems and develop mutual understanding. The statement of principles of relationship between physicians and hospitals that emerged from these meetings and was subsequently endorsed by both the AMA and the AHA in 1953 was equitable and realistic.[5] A clear and positive statement of the ethics of the salaried physician was presented to the Judicial Council of the AMA in November, 1952.

When the AMA-AHA joint committee first met, the primary subject on the agenda was the relationship of the salaried physician to the medical profession, the specialty boards, and the hospital, and the AMA code of ethics. The committee realized, however, that this was only part of the problem of hospital-physician relationships. The statement also dealt with the necessity for a close relationship between the medical staff and the governing board of the hospital. We agreed that financial relationships between the physician and hospitals should be developed at the local level, based upon local conditions and needs, so long as neither physician, hospital, or patient was exploited.

Unfortunately, the 1953 AMA-AHA agreement was short-lived. The unilateral actions of some of the hospital-based specialty societies and a number of the state medical societies prompted the AMA House of Delegates, in December, 1959, to state that the AMA stood by the policy adopted in 1951 and not the position agreed to jointly with the AHA in 1953 and reaffirmed by the AHA in the middle of 1959.[6] This action might have been

5. "American Medical Association and the American Hospital Association," *Hospitals* 27 (August, 1953), 79.
6. "AMA Acts on Hospital-Physician Relations," (Retraction of 1953 position), *Hospitals* 33 (December 16, 1959), 17–19.

expected, for individual specialists and hospital-based specialty organizations who disagreed with the 1953 statement had simply continued to go their own way, using whatever statement or decision that best fitted their purpose.

Now, almost thirty years later, the attitudes of organized medicine and its specialties toward salary have changed. In August, 1982, the Federal Trade Commission forbade the AMA to "interfere with either the amount or the form of compensation provided a member in exchange for his or her professional services, in contracts with entities offering physician services to the public." The AMA Principle of Ethics has been changed and physicians may now be employed by hospitals on salary.

THE BATTLE OF THE ATTORNEYS GENERAL OPINIONS

Opinions of state attorneys general also figured in the continuing controversy about physicians on salary. I became involved in such opinions in both Connecticut and Iowa. The activities leading to the opinions arose from the same pressures and issues already described.

Much of the activity of attorneys general nationwide dated from the appearance in 1949 of "A Study Relating to the Corporate Practice of Medicine in the United States," by Edwin J. Holman, an attorney on the staff of the Bureau of Legal Medicine and Legislation of the AMA.[7] His report undoubtedly played a role in the development of the Hess Report. Its basic thesis was that, if a hospital were to employ a physician and charge for his or her services, or if a medical school were to collect professional fees for the services of its salaried professors, then it would be engaging in the illegal corporate practice of medicine. When a specific case arose, the usual procedure was for some official body to request an opinion of the state attorney general.

A number of such opinions appeared within a relatively short time, but the result was inconclusive. Attorneys General in Connecticut and North Carolina ruled that employment of salaried physicians was not illegal, but in Colorado, Florida, Idaho, Iowa, Ohio, Virginia, Michigan, and West Virginia, the attorneys general ruled that arrangements involving charges by hospitals for medical services were unlawful. In most states, there was no change in existing patterns regardless of the legal opinions expressed, apparently because courts and legislatures were not thought the proper bodies to resolve complex problems of professional relationships in medical and hospital care. This attitude was reinforced by

7. E. J. Holman, "A Study Relating to the Corporate Practice of Medicine in the United States," Bureau of Legal Medicine and Legislation, American Medical Association 1949, pp. 1–50.

what happened in Iowa, where a long and bitter trial resulted in a lower-court decision against hospitals charging and collecting for pathology and radiology services. As far as I know, this was the only instance in which an attorney general's opinion came to trial, and the result wasn't particularly satisfying to anyone.

THE IOWA TRIAL

The Iowa trial started in November, 1952, and continued throughout the decade. There were two main issues. One involved an attempt to change the method of reimbursement for professional services, such as pathology and radiology, from Blue Cross to Blue Shield. The second was an effort to conform to a relatively rigid ruling by the attorney general of Iowa that hospitals were engaged in the corporate practice of medicine if they had individual physicians on salary or with some other arrangement that did not conform to the practices of other physicians. Actually, no specialty physician was on salary in any Iowa voluntary hospital. A percentage of the gross income, with the hospital billing for services, was the common arrangement. Nothing was ever said about the salaried physicians in the University Hospital or in state or federal tuberculosis, mental, Public Health Service, or military institutions.

Societies of pathologists, radiologists, anesthesiologists, and the AMA strongly supported the position of the Iowa attorney general, as did the state medical society. The Iowa Hospital Association opposed the ruling and was supported by the AHA. It was, in microcosm, the same controversy that had occupied the Hess Committee, the Judicial Council of the AMA, and the hospital-based specialists.

In November, 1954, E. Dwight Barnett and I (as chairman of the AHA Council on Professional Practice) for the AHA, and Dwight Murray and Walter Martin for the AMA, along with staff from both organizations, met with the Iowa representatives to try to get an agreement. The only result was a relatively innocuous, hopeful recommendation that they "go back to taw," in the words of Dr. Martin, and work it out at the local level. But no one believed that this could be done. The medical representatives knew that they had an opinion in their favor—why make any effort to change it?

Eventually, the Iowa Hospital Association decided to challenge the opinion in court. I was consulted and agreed with this action. I was horrified, however, at the argument the hospitals adopted on the advice of a former senior member of the AHA staff who was a doctor of medicine, a lawyer, and a hospital administrator. He told the Iowa hospital representatives to maintain that radiology and pathology (with the exception, perhaps, of surgical pathology) were not really medicine. The personal physician was the real doctor: the radiologist, for example, only took x-rays, looked at some shadows, and gave an opinion to the personal physician. The physician then made the diagnosis based on the patient's history, physical examination, the descriptive findings of the radiologist and the pathologist, and perhaps some additional studies. Thus, only the personal physician was diagnosing and treating the patient. I considered this a glib, specious, and indefensible approach that would only infuriate pathologists, radiologists, and their colleagues.

My doubts were correct. The trial went on for a considerable period with weeks and months between sessions. I had no more to do with it until the hospital representatives asked me to appear as an expert witness in their behalf. I learned that they were having trouble finding doctors to testify. Time after time, they lined one up only to get a telephone call or a telegram at the last moment saying that he or she would be unable to attend. We had little doubt that they were bowing to pressure from their peers. I was willing to appear for the hospital association, but by the time they asked me there were two rather substantial obstacles. First, I refused to be party to the position that pathologists and radiologists were not practicing medicine. Second, I had become president-elect of the AHA and was afraid that if I appeared the association might be considered to have entered the legal controversy officially.

The Iowa hospital representatives and their attorneys came to New Haven, and went over their arguments with John Tilson, counsel for the CHA. They agreed that the argument that pathologists and radiologists were not real doctors was unsound, and they abandoned it. I then went to Chicago to discuss the overall strategy with Edwin Crosby, executive director of the AHA. As I expected, Dr. Crosby did not approve of the AHA appearing to be involved, and I am not sure that he ever forgave me for going to Iowa. However, I felt that the Iowa hospitals were in trouble and that I might be of value to them. I hoped that I could make it clear that I was speaking for myself and not for the AHA.

It was an interesting but fruitless experience. The judge ruled in favor of the attorney general's interpretations. He also emphasized that radiology and pathology were the practice of medicine and that financial arrangements should reflect this in such a manner that the hospitals could not be considered to be in the corporate practice of medicine. Afterward, there was considerable debate as to whether the Iowa hospitals should appeal, but it was finally decided instead to develop compromise legislation. Representatives of the Iowa Hospital Association, the Iowa Medical Society, and the Iowa State Board of Medical Examiners drafted a proposed physician-hospital agreement, which was then approved by the Iowa Hospital Association and the Iowa State Medical Society. This agreement was enacted virtually verbatim by the Iowa State Legislature in the spring of 1957.

It is still difficult to evaluate the results of the vast expenditures of money, emotion, and time that went into this battle. The shift of radiology and pathology services from Blue Cross to Blue Shield may have stimulated the specialty societies in their final negotiations on Medicare in 1965, which included hospital-based specialties under Part B instead of Part A (see chapter 11). There were however, no demonstrable changes in the professional status of radiologists and pathologists and no substantial differences in the relative incomes of the medical specialists and the hospital. And, although the hospitals and the hospital-based specialists in Iowa were relatively satisfied after the dust had settled, the American College of Radiology and one of its leaders, Harry Garland, indicated dismay with the Iowa agreements and the subsequent legislative action. The college published criticisms of the decision and proposed further legislative action.

Following the Iowa trial, the issues of physicians on salary decreased in importance, as did ethics as a subject for state legislative action. Finally, in 1984, the Iowa legislature once again changed the Iowa code to permit hospitals to employ specialty physicians under any form of compensation mutually agreed upon. (The 1982 FTC action described earlier may have had something to do with this change.)

The Iowa trial generated unexpected repercussions a few years later. I was an AHA appointee to the Joint Commission on the Accreditation of Hospitals from 1955 to 1964. The chairmanship of the commission rotates each year through the several member organizations, and the senior member of the organization due to have the chairmanship is usually elected. Near the end of my nine years on the commission, I was the senior AHA member and was in line for the post. The morning of the JCAH meeting, several of the AMA representatives, who were all respected friends of mine, took me aside and, with some embarrassment, informed me that the AMA group had decided to oppose my being elected as chairman. The reason was my participation for the hospitals in the Iowa trial—they believed that AMA members throughout the country would resent my being the commission chairman. They expected anger and argument from me and were thus surprised when I promptly said that I would vote against my own election.

My reasons for giving up the position were relatively simple. It was prestigious, but it involved additional time in Chicago. Also, a good presiding officer encourages discussion and is restricted in expressing his or her own opinions. I knew that the JCAH's contribution to the quality of care in hospitals was vitally important and that the commission needed as much support as possible from both physicians and hospitals. Virtually every meeting of the AMA House of Delegates produced one or more resolutions, from state medical societies or some individual members of the house, criticizing some aspect, regulation, or procedure of the JCAH. Constant vigilance was necessary to preserve the authority and the contribution of the commission, which was (and still is) one of the most important bodies concerned with the quality of health care. I knew that my being chairman would be an unnecessary handicap for the commission. So another commission member got the post, and I possess the unique honor of being the only potential chairman of the JCAH who was spurned.

RADIOLOGY

After all the arguments, correspondence, challenges, interpretations, and clarifications of the rulings on salaried physicians that took place in the 1940s and 1950s, the radiologists opened fire again in February, 1958. A policy statement adopted by the Board of Chancellors of the American College of Radiology declared that it was unethical for any radiologist to enter into relationships with hospitals, medical schools, or other corporations in which his or her services were provided for a fee payable to the corporation. It reiterated that radiology should not be covered in hospital service insurance contracts. It also implied that punitive action would be taken toward radiologists who did not comply with the policy.

By 1958, I had graduated from being an assistant hospital administrator, uttering shrill and indignant cries from the sidelines, to the executive directorship of a university teaching hospital with salaried physicians in all types of specialties. I had also been chairman of the AHA Council on Professional Practice and president of the AHA. I had had constructive (although sometimes laborious and extended) exchanges with the officers and staff of the AMA and the specialty organizations and had developed increasing respect for and friendship with their leaders as individuals. But it seemed that any agreement—no matter how formally approved—became ephemeral when vocal members of the organization wanted to change it. And the disagreements always seemed to be related to salary and economics.

The radiologists' policy statement resulted in my sending off another round of correspondence and writing another detailed article, which recited again the pronouncements and rulings of the AMA board and its Judicial Council. This was published early in 1960, accompanied by correspondence between me and Vincent W. Archer, president of the American College of Radiology, concerning its policy statements.[8] I asked Dr. Archer a number of specific questions:

1. Was patient care inferior when radiologists were on salary?
2. Did salaried physicians in the armed services, the Public Health Services, or the Veterans Administration provide lower-grade care because they were salaried? What about salaried faculty in medical schools?
3. Was the quality of service and patient care rendered by radiologists employed by hospitals, medical schools, or governmental agencies inferior to that of a radiologist employed by another radiologist?

Dr. Archer's answer to all of the above questions was yes. He continued, "such a radiologist employed by another radiologist would be considered ethical." As might be guessed, the extensive correspondence and debate convinced no one, and little change occurred in most of the major institutions thoughout the country. Many of their radiologists—particularly those in the large university hospitals—were on salary, but others were on a fee-for-service basis or received a percentage of the gross income. Percentage of net income raised too much controversy over what should be included in costs, and leasing arrangements were frequently insecure because of legal complications of the nonprofit status of the hospital. I am not sure why further attempts were made to resolve the disagreement, but perhaps it was partly due to my continued challenges and my accusations that the radiologists were confusing ethics and economics. Whatever the reason, I was completely amazed when, in December, 1960, Harry Garland asked me if I would be willing to help work out a statement of relationship between hospitals and radiologists.

Dr. Garland was the radiologist-in-chief at the San Francisco County Hospital (now the San Francisco General Hospital) and a professor of radiology at Stanford Medical School. Both my wife, Parnie, and I had been his medical students when we rotated through the San Francisco County Hospital. I respected him as a radiologist and as a teacher, and apparently he thought well of me. Dr. Garland was a stormy petrel in medical and radiological circles in San Francisco and had gradually become active in the American College of Radiology. By the time he got in touch with me he was on his way to becoming its president. I had been president of the AHA and was now beginning to gain a reputation as an elder statesman. Dr. Garland wanted us to try to work something out personally and then to involve a liaison committee of the American

8. A. Snoke, "Financial Relationships between Radiologists and Hospitals," *Hospitals* 34, 2–3 (January 16, February 1, 1960), 38–42, 63–68; 43–45, 106–07.

College of Radiology and the AHA. I was delighted. I knew that he was a tough and ardent advocate of the independent practice of radiology, but I also considered him fair and honest, and he was respected by his colleagues.

We met unofficially over the next year or so and worked on a joint statement. At our first meeting, Dr. Parnie and I met with Dr. Garland and William Stronach, executive secretary of the American College of Radiology, and developed our ideas of how we might produce a joint statement. An exchange of letters and consultations with our colleagues on both sides took place, and we got together again in October, 1961. I had ruptured a spinal disc on a canoe trip that summer and was still trying to escape from the neurosurgeons. I lay on the bed in a room in the Plaza Hotel in New York, while Harry Garland paced the room and Dr. Parnie took notes. We thrashed out a pretty good preliminary statement. The result was a meeting of an ad hoc committee of the American College of Radiology and the AHA on principles of hospital-radiologist relationships in November. We agreed on the statement and recommended it for approval by our boards. By February, 1962, the proposed principles had been transmitted to the AHA board of trustees, which approved it contingent upon its approval by the American College of Radiology.[9] Dr. Garland and his associate at the college, Dr. Wachowski, took the statement to his executive board, which also approved it. However, they apparently thought that it needed to go to a larger, more representative group, the Board of Chancellors. This body refused to approve it unless certain changes were made.

The same attitude had been encountered in the AHA, but the ad hoc committee and the board insisted that the original statement had been developed in good faith by both sides and that it should and could not be altered. The American College of Radiology, however, would not accept the joint statement, particularly because some members of the Board of Chancellors still insisted that salary was unethical and would have nothing to do with any statement that said otherwise.

So the result of this final effort was again nothing. Today it is interesting to note that many radiologists in medical centers are still on salary, but they are now employed in the medical school rather than the hospital. In New Haven they have been shifted from the hospital to the medical school, but the radiology department charges its professional fees separately at rates comparable to the other radiologists in the community—substantially above fees accepted by Medicare. Presumably they are ethical today.

9. AHA Board of Trustees, "Hospital-Radiologist Relationships," February 1, 1962.

ANESTHESIOLOGY

The anesthetists and their state and national organizations had the same stormy relationship with hospitals as did the radiologists from the early 1940s to the 1960s. They fought against any type of salary and insisted on charging fees, using the Hess Report and its various modifications, as well as statements of the AMA Judicial Council when they seemed to support their point of view, and ignoring them when they did not. The anesthesia groups took on everyone from the large teaching hospitals to the full-time professors of anesthesiology and prestigious medical schools to poor, young physicians who were starting out in anesthesia and needed their specialty board examinations.

I became aware of the problems of the young anesthetists in the early 1950s. Dr. Hampton, the chief of anesthesia, told me he was having difficulty getting young physician anesthetists on salary. They were hesistant to join the hospital on salary because they would then be considered unethical and would be prevented from taking their specialty board examinations.

I found out that there was an unpublicized, interlocking mechanism by which organized anesthesiology could deter or prevent young anesthetists from going on salary. It took me a year to dig out the facts, because no one wanted to talk or write for the record. But I finally discovered that the American Board of Anesthesiology required anyone wishing to take the specialty board examinations to obtain his certification had to be a member of the American Society of Anesthesiologists. This organization, in turn, required that its members belong to a state society of anesthesiologists. The Connecticut Society of Anesthesiologists had a requirement for membership that the applicant not be on salary. As a result, a young anesthesiologist on salary in Grace-New Haven would not be eligible to apply for examination by his specialty board.

Each of these organizations piously disclaimed any responsibility for the rules and regulations of the others. I pointed out that they were preventing young doctors from obtaining specialty board approval because their interlocking rules were based on forms of remuneration rather than competence. I started this campaign alone in Connecticut. Later, I became acquainted with three prominent medical anesthesiologists, Henry Beecher of MGH, Donald Proctor of Johns Hopkins, and Austin Lamont of the University of Pennsylvania, who were also battling organized anesthesiology on the principle of salary. Together we continued to challenge the organizations from the hospitals' point of view and to publicize their prohibitory system. We finally enlisted allies who put pressure on the American Board of Anesthesiology. The AMA Council on Medical Education and Hospitals, the American College of Surgeons, and, through Robin Buerki, the Allied Medical Specialty Boards all took up cudgels. Finally the American Board of Anesthesiology grudgingly acquiesced and removed the requirement that an applicant had to be a member of the American Society of Anesthesiology before taking the specialty board examinations.

I was never happy with my long drawn-out debates with the organized anesthesiology bodies, for I respected the anesthetists as individuals. Many of the advances in surgery in our hospital would not have been possible without the careful attention of Nicholas Greene and his associates to the necessity for extended periods of anesthesia during prolonged operations. I am not sure who won the economic battles in the long run, but I cannot resist citing the Association of American Medical Colleges (AAMC) *1985–86 Report on Medical School Faculty Salaries*, which reports the compensation base and supplements of full-time faculty with M.D. degrees in private and public medical schools in the Northeast, September, 1985. The highest mean annual income for instructors was $98,900 for anesthesiologists. The next highest figures were $94,000 for orthopedic surgery and $81,000 for neurosurgery. Radiologists' mean annual income was only $55,000—a $15,000 increase over the previous year.

PHYSICAL MEDICINE AND INHALATION THERAPY

Sometime after becoming administrator of Grace-New Haven, I discovered that the medical director of the department of physical therapy was an orthopedic specialist with little interest in or knowledge of physical medicine. He admitted that he was no specialist in this field and had no objection to my searching for a physiatrist to head the department. In 1951, we invited Thomas Hines to join the hospital. It seemed clear that, as a specialist in a little-known field, he should have a full-time salary.

Dr. Hines was not only administrator of the department but also a consultant, helping physicians who were referring patients for physical therapy. Before he arrived, many of them merely sent their patients to the department with a prescription blank reading "Rx: Physical Therapy," leaving the physical therapists to decide what treatment was needed. (The situation has not changed much over the past forty years. A physical therapist recently told me that she had received a prescription blank from a physician that said only "Help!") It became Dr. Hines's responsibility to review the situation with the patient and the doctor and prescribe a course of treatment. He followed the patients through therapy and discharged them when he and the physician felt it appropriate. Nevertheless, it took years for the physicians in the community to recognize Dr. Hines's value. If he had had to develop a referral practice and derive his income on a fee-for-service basis, he would have starved.

The same situation occurred when we learned that patients who were receiving oxygen or inhalation therapy were being cared for primarily by the nurses or orderlies. Few of the staff members knew anything about a Bird Respirator, and orderlies or nurses put patients in oxygen tents or introduced nasal catheters when ordered by the attending physician. We once almost lost a patient because the tube was put down the wrong orifice, and occasionally a patient got bluer in an oxygen tent because an orderly had replaced one used-up oxygen tank with another. It seemed clear that inhalation therapy needed professional direction, but to attract an expert to train the technicians and be available for consultation in the many complicated situations required money. Donald Egan came to the hospital in 1956. Again, he could never have made his living on a referral or private fee basis. It was perfectly logical to put him on salary.

Both situations illustrate problems that the hospital administrator and an informed medical board can solve when the need is clear. Together we recognized that the sensible—indeed the only—mechanism by which certain essential personnel could be employed was salary. Without it, these two experts would never have entered the medical scene in New Haven. To consider them unethical because they were salaried would be ridiculous and would have deprived many patients of crucial services. Individual physicians on the hospital staff agreed—their organizations did not!

PATHOLOGY

For various reasons, my experience with pathologists, both individual and organizational, was much less adversarial than it was with radiologists and anesthesiologists. I must admit to profound prejudice favoring pathologists. The dean of the Stanford Medical School when I started as a medical student there (and the dean at its predecessor when my father received his M.D. in 1906) was William Ophuls, a renowned pathologist. At SMH, the dean of the Medical School was a Nobel Prize winner, George Whipple, a pathologist and one of the most dedicated and able scientists and humanists I have ever known. And in New Haven the professor of pathology was Milton Winternitz, who was dean of the Yale Medical School during its renaissance. All these men were the finest in teaching, research, and patient care. (It may not have been coincidental that all were on salary but all were tolerant of a variety of financial arrangements.)

Pathology is not a simple, straightforward specialty. Autopsy and tissue pathology were early subdivisions, but even in 1930 clinical chemistry, bacteriology, hematology, and clinical microscopy were part of what was to become the specialty of clinical pathology. Laboratories were usually directed by physicians, but many were headed by Ph.D.s in chemistry or bacteriology. In all three medical centers with which I was associated, the laboratory services were divided into autopsy and tissue pathology, headed by traditional anatomical and tissue pathologists, and clinical laboratory subdivisions headed by internists, pediatricians, or Ph.D.s who were most interested in the services that were related to their own specialties.

In New Haven, I found serious administrative and service problems in the pathology department. There was one autopsy and tissue pathology department, and it was primarily oriented to teaching and research. Clinical pathology was quite fragmented, consisting of at least two blood chemistry labs, two bacteriology labs, three clinical microscopy and hematology labs, and separate labs for hemolytic streptococci, blood iodides, and other specific examinations, plus the individual ward service laboratories for the medical students and resident staff.

This contrasted sharply with the typical laboratory such as I found in the Grace Hospital (which was then combining with the New Haven Hospital). I was fortunate that Charles Bartlett, a retired professor of pathology at Yale Medical School, was in charge. Dr. Bartlett and his successor, Levin Waters, encouraged me to press for a consolidation of the many specialized laboratories in the New Haven unit and eventually in the hospital as a whole. Dean Long of the Yale Medical School told me that a colleague, Gerald T. Evans, had started consolidating the laboratories at the University of Minnesota teaching hospital in 1939. I visited him and then began patiently persuading the individual academic entrepreneurs in New Haven to combine their activities. The first head of our consolidated laboratory was a Ph.D. bacteriologist and mycologist, Lenore Haley, who also started a medical technology program. As the laboratory activities and responsibilities grew, both Dr. Haley and I recognized the value of finding an M.D. clinical pathologist to be the director. We invited David Seligson of Philadelphia to visit and consult. He gave us a politely devastating description of our inadequacies. The obvious response was to invite him to come to New Haven and develop a new department of clinical pathology in the hospital and the medical school. He accepted the challenge in 1958.

The addition of Dr. Seligson in clinical pathology led to improvement in the variety of procedures: greater accuracy and dependability in the laboratory analyses, the attraction and retention of able counterparts in the various subspecialties, and increased economy of operations. As with the other chiefs of service, Dr. Seligson was salaried, and I caused him considerable embarrassment by extolling the superlative service and economical operation of the department in my continuing arguments with the AMA, the hospital-based specialists, and in the battle on Medicare. The patients benefitted from the dependable and rapid service available to them and their attending physicians, and the hospital gained because we could keep our costs to them and to the third party payers at a reasonable level.

6

The Teaching Hospital

The teaching hospital has been the basis of most of my education in hospital and health care administration for the past fifty years. Part of this education has resulted from what these hospitals have done—part from what many have not.

During the early years of my career, I shared a snobbish sense of superiority with many others like me over the preeminence of university teaching hospitals. Most of my professors and resident staff colleagues had studied at Johns Hopkins, Yale, Harvard, Columbia, Cornell, Penn, Chicago, Washington University at St. Louis, and the University of California. I went east in 1936 primarily because I wanted to see for myself whether the eastern medical establishment was really the mecca of medicine. I wanted to be able to return to the West Coast no longer feeling that I had to genuflect whenever anyone mentioned Baltimore, Boston, New Haven, or New York. Undoubtedly I also wanted to assume that same spurious mantle of superiority by dropping the name of some eastern institution in discussions with my West Coast colleagues. During ten years in Rochester and twenty-two in New Haven, accompanied by increasing activity in the AHA, I learned the weaknesses as well as the strengths of the university teaching hospitals and the value of the non-university teaching hospital. I also learned that there were no geographical boundaries to medical excellence.

From the 1920s through the 1940s, university hospitals or institutions with close affiliations to medical schools attracted most of the top students for internships and residencies and were generally acknowledged as the leaders in medical and hospital care. The resident staff in these hospitals usually had a great deal of responsibility for the care of patients. The combination of faculty and resident staff not only stimulated local community hospitals to improve care, but also gradually extended their standards throughout their regions. They also provided leadership in regional and state hospital associations.

Most of the teaching hospitals had departmental chiefs of service— usually professors in the university or medical school, frequently on salary, although sometimes on one of various types of fee-for-service reimbursement. Their offices, laboratories, and clinical practices were usually located in the hospital or medical center. The importance of full-time chiefs of service was first emphasized by Winford H. Smith, director of Johns Hopkins Hospital, in his 1917 consultation report to Yale University and the New Haven Hospital. He wrote, in the most unflattering terms, that Yale had a second- or third-rate medical school and hospital, which would not materially improve until it adopted a program employing full-time salaried faculty and chiefs of service. Yale did so in 1918, and many of the other major hospitals in the country soon followed suit.

By the time I became associated with the administration of teaching hospitals in 1937, a number of other significant changes had taken place. One of these was the shift in the nature of the "teaching material." Stanford, for example, housed its ward and teaching service in the old Lane Hospital Division; private patients were in the newer Stanford Hospital Unit. Patients at Lane and at the San Francisco County Hospital provided medical education and experience for students and residents. At the county hospitals of San Francisco, Alameda County, and Los Angeles, interns and residents were fairly promptly given major responsibility for the care of indigent patients. More carefully supervised services were provided by residents at Stanford-Lane, but all of the teaching was done with patients housed in wards containing twenty to forty beds. The wards at Bellevue Hospital in New York City and Cook County Hospital in Chicago also provided important teaching resources for most of their cities' medical schools. In all these hospitals indigent patients were expected to be teaching material in return for medical care without charge.

The University of Rochester and Strong Memorial Hospital started out with a similar philosophy, substantially assisted by a far-sighted health officer, George Goler, who arranged for the Rochester Municipal Hospital (RMH) to be built in 1926 as part of the construction of the new (SMH). The original plans called for a full-time, salaried faculty to provide care and teach in both the RMH and SMH which would house what were termed "service" (instead of "ward") patients. Professional fees were not to be charged to service patients, and all rooms were to have no more than four beds.

The original plan proved unrealistic in regard to the class of patient to be cared for in SMH. Patients who could afford to pay demanded care from the prestigious medical school faculty. When the hospital was completed in 1926, it had one-bed, two-bed, and four-bed rooms, and all the patients, whether service or private, in multi-bed accommodations in SMH were considered "teaching material." This attitude gradually led to the philosophy that all patients, regardless of their accomodations, were considered available for teaching. New Haven Hospital, the primary teaching hospital for Yale Medical School, went through the same evolution from larger wards in the older buildings to newer construction with only one-bed, two-bed, or four-bed rooms. However, it took longer for the hospital and the Yale Medical School to accept the principle that teaching could be done with private patients.

This shift came about not because of any sudden change of philosophy but because of inescapable economic realities. As more and more patients had Blue Cross, Blue Shield, commercial insurance, and Medicare, they could afford private or semi-private care. The original reservoir of patients for teaching shrank remarkably. In addition, the faculty realized that the resident staff was of great assistance in the care of their private patients. The presence of medical students plus the teaching atmosphere thus contributed to improved professional care. Private patients were rare who refused to be involved in the teaching when it was properly explained—and especially once faculty learned to hold their clinical discussion away from the patient's bedside.

Although medical students' teaching material now usually includes both paying and nonpaying patients, some medical schools still build their programs around low-income patients and hospitals. I question this philosophy, not only because of the obvious financial advantages of having private patients, but also because the atmosphere and the attitude toward patients in the institution is important in training. I felt that the atmosphere and patient care in both Rochester and New Haven were superior because the faculty, the attending staff, and the patients came from a wide variety of economic and social backgrounds. This attitude admittedly cannot be easily quantified. It is interesting, however, that lists of the ten "best hospitals" that periodically appear include primarily hospitals which have a strong community physician presence and in which private patients are part of the undergraduate and postgraduate educational programs. Another change that took place was the expansion of internship and residency programs into hospitals not directly affiliated with universities or medical schools. Originally, the university teaching hospital was part of a medical center in which teaching, research, and service all played a part. As medical specialties evolved, so did the resident staff; most of whom eventually left to go into practice. Although some remained in the medical center or its immediate community, many went to other hospitals where they eventually became specialists and chiefs of service. Thus, university hospitals trained their own competition. The larger of these institutions began to develop internship and residency programs of their own and became teaching hospitals and respected competitors of the university hospitals for the care of specialized conditions. Thoracic and cardiac surgery, neurosurgery, oncology, cardiovascular disease, hematology, endocrinology, and the like have now become accepted specialties in many institutions other than university hospitals. Affiliations with medical schools have been made and rotation or sponsorship of student or resident education developed.

When I first started in administration in SMH, I was introduced to the University Hospital Executive Council (UHEC), an informal group of chief executives of the teaching hospitals of the universities of Rochester, Western Reserve in Cleveland, Chicago, Michigan, Indiana, Iowa, Wisconsin, and Minnesota, which met once or twice a year. When I came to New Haven in 1946, I felt young and alone, because there were no local administrators (except for those in the large Hartford Hospital) with whom I could discuss problems. So I invited my counterparts in hospital administration at several eastern universities (plus their deans of medicine and vice presidents for medical affairs, where such positions existed) to a meeting in New Haven. Representatives from MGH-Harvard, Columbia-Presbyterian, New York Hospital-Cornell, the University of Pennsylvania Medical School and Hospital, and Johns Hopkins Hospital and Medical School attended. When SMH and Lakeside Hospital (Western Reserve) heard about this group, they asked to be included. We formed the informal Council of Teaching Hospitals—similar to the Midwestern UHEC. Subsequently, the AAMC formally adopted the name of the Council of Teaching Hospitals (COTH) for its teaching hospitals division, belatedly acknowledging our group as the original council of teaching hospitals in its discussion paper of April, 1984. (My friends, however, preferred to term it the Poison Ivy League.)

A FINANCIAL CRISIS

My first years in New Haven were a real postgraduate course in hospital and health administration. Not only was I the CEO of a major teaching institution, with all the attendant responsibilities, but I also arrived during a crisis in the hospital's financial relationship with Yale University and its medical school. After this traumatic introduction, I became involved in governance, administration, and cost control while I studied relationships between various types of institutions, reimbursement rates for all types of patients, the role of the resident staff in service and hospital costs, and the responsibilities of the teaching hospital to the community, to its neighbors, and to the state.

The immediate crisis that faced me upon my arrival had to do with the fact that the New Haven Hospital had been receiving from Yale University an annual cash subsidy of up to $206,000 a year to meet its operating deficit. The new hospital board believed that this subsidy should be increased. Yale University felt equally strongly that the subsidy should be reduced or discontinued. The future of the Yale Medical School was also in jeopardy.

For some reason, this crisis was kept a deep secret. I knew nothing of it when I arrived in April, 1946, and George Darling knew nothing of it before his appointment in August, 1946, as the university's director of medical affairs. Upon learning of the problem, he immediately told President Seymour that he had not come to New Haven to preside over the demise of the Yale Medical School. Meanwhile, I discovered, after investigating the financial situation in great detail, that, on top of the annual cash subsidy, Yale was also providing approximately $300,000 in laboratory, x-ray, pathology, and other services, for which the hospital received the income. The total subsidy was thus approximately $500,000 a year. But no member of either corporation was aware of these figures (the equivalent of $2.5 million in 1986 dollars)—and no one seemed to be aware that the hospital owned the entire block upon which had been built half of the medical school and the two major patient units. All the university buildings on the site would revert to the hospital at the end of a ninety-nine-year-lease!

There must have been some strategic reason not to publicize the university's concern about the fate of the medical school. I am continually surprised, even now, at how many of those who were presumably in the confidence of the administration have greeted my tale of the medical school's jeopardy with incredulity. The records exist, however—they were discovered years later by a graduate student preparing a thesis on the School of Nursing.[1] I am also still amazed at the hospital board's support of its young administrator when he disagreed with a report from a prestigious consulting firm that recommended the cash subsidy be

1. Sr. Dorothy A. Sheehan, "A Social Origin of American Nursing and its Movement into the University: A Microscopic Approach," Ph.D. Diss. New York University School of Education, 1980.

increased. But after careful analysis and interminable negotiations, Dr. Darling, Dean Long, and I developed a five-year program to eliminate that cash subsidy and to have the hospital assume the service expenses. This required persuading the Connecticut state legislature to enact legislation stipulating that the state and local communities would pay hospital costs for patients who were the responsibility of the welfare departments. Welfare patients made up 20–25 percent of the patient population at Grace-New Haven. The final agreement also required the medical school to abandon its demand that the hospital maintain more than 250 teaching ward beds and start teaching with semi-private and private patients, who had long been overcharged, on the Robin Hood principle, to make up for the losses incurred in the care of low-income patients. The 1952 agreement formally stated that the hospital would furnish teaching beds only to the extent of its financial ability. It also provided for the block owned by the hospital to be divided so that each partner could own its buildings and the land beneath.

The reduction of the university financial and service subsidy, the clarification of ownership of land and buildings, and the elimination of the requirement for a specific number of ward beds for teaching were great successes, probably accomplished because of the mutual respect and friendship among Darling, Long, and myself. It was, of course, satisfying that the university stopped considering cutting back the medical school program to two years.

At a meeting of the Board of Permanent Officers of the Medical School some years later, the new dean reported to the board and to President Whitney Griswold that, although the medical school's appropriation from the university had been frozen for a number of years, it had still been able to increase its budget by half a million dollars and increase faculty salaries. Everyone applauded. I waited to hear how this miracle had been accomplished, but nothing more was said. President Griswold congratulated the dean and everyone was so pleased that I decided not to remind the board that the half a million had come out of the hospital staff's blood, sweat, and tears, and the pocketbooks of taxpayers and patients, who were still being overcharged substantially. It was not until years later that I learned of an additional factor that had contributed to the medical school's financial health. When George Darling had come to Yale in 1946, grants were beginning to make up a substantial portion of the school's income. But the grants did not provide for overhead, and each recipient prepared his or her own salary scale for assistants, technicians, and other staff on the research project. As the research funds grew, the university and the school were under increasing pressure to hire staff to administer the grants and maintain the space required. Personnel problems were also developing because of the varying salary and benefit scales. Dr. Darling patiently worked with the many independent faculty entrepreneurs to develop a single standard for salaries and benefits. And, of more long-ranging significance, he convinced foundations and the government to recognize overhead as a legitimate component of research grants.

BALANCING ACTS

Teaching, research, and service have for years been the combined mission of the university teaching hospital. Inevitably, there are battles over priorities, the outcomes of which often depend upon the dean of the medical school, the available funds, the attitude toward academic promotion, and the perceived needs of the community. These factors, of course, are not constant. In my early years in administration, teaching and patient care were essentially interdependent, but research was assuming ever-increasing importance. By the time I came to Yale, research was becoming top priority. This is not difficult to understand. Grants from the National Institute of Health (NIH) were a major source of income for medical schools, and research publications were essential for grants and promotion.

I was often told by the dean and the chairmen of the clinical departments that promotion was based upon superlative performance in two, but not necessarily all three, areas of teaching, research, and patient care. But when I sat in on discussions of promotion or tenure, the primary emphasis seemed always to be upon the list of publications. "Publish or perish" was and often still is a basic fact of life in academia. The practical aspect cannot be overlooked; research begets research grants, which in turn produce more papers and more possibilities for promotion and tenure, and also attracts gifted assistants. Publication also brings prominence, visiting professorships, appointments to study committees, lectures, and site visits—all of which enhance one's reputation and make life exciting. But, back home at the hospital, the students have to be taught and patients cared for. I used to tell the dean that he needed three sets of faculty—one going, one returning, and one tending to business at home.

The university hospital administrator has problems with this type of senior medical staff environment. A stable, high census of patients is necessary to pay for the budgeted staffing pattern. A sudden, sharp drop in the census on the surgical or medical divisions is disconcerting at first, but soon it is recognized as a signal that certain specialties or clinical

research organizations are meeting. Most of the faculty go to these meetings to read papers, listen, exchange information, or seek academic
advancement. It is nevertheless important for the faculty and the administration of both the medical school and the hospital to recognize the
necessity of maintaining an appropriate patient census.

As a result of the recent decrease in federal financial support to
medical schools for additional enrollment and grants, a marked change in
the attitudes of medical school faculty and administration has taken place.
Paying patients and income from professional fees are now given greater
priority, for this type of income is necessary to replace government
support. From the hospital's point of view, it is, of course, helpful for the
medical school faculty to recognize the need for continuing high census.
But an unfortunate byproduct in some medical centers has been competition and friction between the full-time medical school faculty and their
community associates. The three-year struggle between town and gown
in New Haven (described in chapter 4) illustrates the need for an administration that can balance the needs of the medical staff, patients,
researchers, and community.

Of major importance is the working relationship between the hospital administrator, the dean of the medical school, and the vice president or
chancellor for health affairs. Administration of a hospital or a medical
school is a full-time responsibility, and only an unusual person can
balance fairly the several components of teaching, research, patient care,
and community. Perhaps this did not pose a serious problem to me
because my being interested in patient care and community service
convinced me that, in providing these services in a fine institution, I was
also providing the best possible laboratory in which the medical school,
the nursing school, and the school of public health could teach and
research.

If the administration of a university hospital demands special
qualities, so does the role of the dean of a medical school. Not the least of
the dean's problems is the aura of omniscience that surrounds the position. The dean's authority and power are not necessarily accepted for long
by his or her associates, but others frequently regard the dean as a
superior being. There is no question that a medical center needs an
academic dean. However, when the medical school and hospital are
owned by one entity (university, county, or state), conflict between the
dean and the hospital administrator is almost inevitable. Because of the
superior aura surrounding the dean, these conflicts often lead to the
hospital administrator's being replaced, demoted, or administratively
emasculated.

Conflict need not prevail, however. A classic example of accord occurred between the smh and the University of Rochester. George Whipple, a pathologist and Nobel laureate, was dean of the medical school; Basil MacLean was director of the hospital. The university considered Dean Whipple the ultimate authority, but he and Dr. MacLean worked as partners and colleagues. As an assistant, I wondered whether this was because they were good friends or because Dr. Whipple respected Dr. MacLean's ability and experience. I learned the answer when, for eighteen months during World War II, I was the acting director of the hospital while Dr. MacLean was in the Surgeon General's office in Washington. My relationship with the dean was exactly the same as Dr. MacLean's. He never interfered with my operation of the hospital, nor did the associate dean, George Berry, who later became dean of Harvard Medical School. George Berry and I argued constantly, primarily over philosophy. I never let him forget his comment that he and the medical school regarded the hospital as just another subdivision of the medical school, like the animal house! Although Berry was indulging in hyperbole, many deans have dominated medical centers at the expense of the hospital's patient care responsibilities and, often, at the expense of the hospital administrator. Thus, when Dean Whipple retired, his successor, Donald Anderson, quickly assumed a number of Dr. MacLean's responsibilities and wanted to take over his office. As a result, Dr. MacLean took one of the many job offers he had repeatedly turned down and became commissioner of hospitals in New York City.

Working relationships between independent institutions, when the two organizations have strong leaders and mutual respect, are excellent examples of cooperation. New York Hospital and Cornell University and Medical School have done well with a joint administrative board. Yale University and the Grace-New Haven Community Hospital worked equally well when George Darling represented the university as its director of medical affairs and I represented the hospital as its director. Today, there are many major university medical centers in which the university, the county, or the state owns both medical school and hospital and has associated with the center a number of allied health science schools—medical, dental, nursing, and pharmacy. In these cases, a vice president for medical or health affairs is almost a necessity. The best structure includes an academic dean for teaching and research, a hospital administrator primarily concerned with people care and management, and a vice president for medical affairs who will allow each to carry out his or her responsibilities and not interfere with the lines of communication and authority. If the vice president also tries to function as the dean of medicine, the hospital administrator risks becoming essentially an institutional superintendent.

AAMC AND THE TEACHING HOSPITALS

Prior to the late 1950s, the Association of American Medical Colleges was essentially a dean's club which met once a year, had a small executive staff, and welcomed about 20 percent of its membership as new deans each year, reflecting the annual turnover. A number of university hospital administrators—particularly Donald Caseley from Illinois and Gerhard Hartman of the University of Iowa—prevailed upon the organization to form a medical school–teaching hospital section. Hartman and Caseley were the first two chairmen, and at their second meeting they asked if I would be the third. Somewhat skeptical of both the AAMC and the new organization of administrators, I asked, "why me?" They answered, "because we need someone who can talk back to the deans." A peculiar but challenging reason. I accepted.

As chairman of the section, I was invited to speak at a plenary session of the AAMC in November, 1959. I titled my talk, "The Teaching Hospital— Its Responsibilities and Conflicts," and emphasized the problem of balancing teaching, research, and service.[2] I used the old example of the three-legged milkmaid's stool to represent the three components of the university teaching hospital and gleefully quoted statements such as that of the professor at Johns Hopkins who wrote that "university departments of pediatrics . . . must be devoted largely to research in human biology rather than to the practical training of individuals, although this may be an important by-product of the activities of the department," and Dean Berry's equation of the hospital with the animal house. I also mentioned a USPHS report on medical schools' needs which seemed to see the teaching hospitals only as providers of medical research beds. The milkmaid's stool example was repeated for a number of years at AAMC meetings—usually referred to as "Snoke's damned milkmaid's stool." One of my prized possessions is a small, appropriately engraved three-legged stool given to me some years later as one of the past chairmen of the teaching group. Now they only present the retired chairman with a gavel.[3]

2. A. Snoke, "The Teaching Hospital—Its Responsibilities and Conflicts," *Journal of Medical Education* 35 (November 3, 1980), 207–13.

3. Although time apparently heals many prejudices: to my pleasure and amazement, the teaching hospital section of the AAMC recently presented John A. D. Cooper, on his retirement as president of the AAMC, with a handsome, engraved, three-legged milkmaid's stool!

Hartman, Caseley, and I did not realize what we were starting with the hospital group. The programs of the teaching hospital section turned out to be better than those of the deans, and within a few years the program of the annual AAMC meeting was as stimulating as those of the other national health-care organizations. The AAMC was substantially reorganized in 1965, following the recommendations of Lowell Coggeshall of Chicago, and the teaching hospital section became an equal division and took a new name, the Council of Teaching Hospitals (COTH).

The formation of the section in 1957–58 and of COTH in 1965 also had repercussions far wider than originally intended. First, the concept of the teaching hospital expanded to include more than just the primary hospital associated with a medical school. Russell A. Nelson, director of Johns Hopkins Hospital, and I were impressed with the contributions of the many other hospitals that not only had major internship and resident staff programs but also were important resources for medical student education. As members of the AAMC planning committee for COTH, we also cited such hospitals as Hartford Hospital in Connecticut, the Rhode Island Hospital in Providence, and the Mary Hitchcock Memorial Hospital in Hanover, New Hampshire, all of which had directors of medical education and were superlative teaching institutions, although not primary university teaching hospitals at that time. From this expanded concept of a teaching hospital, the COTH membership grew from less than 100 hospitals primarily associated with a medical school to an enrollment of 432 in 1982–83. An unexpected financial dividend may have also occurred from the expansion. Fifteen of the thirty-eight hospitals in Connecticut are now classified as teaching hospitals and are members of COTH. In 1984–85, these fifteen hospitals received substantially higher DRG payments because of their classification.

COSTS OF TEACHING HOSPITALS

Financial relationships between teaching hospitals and medical schools vary greatly, depending upon each partner's cost of operation, income from tuition, services, and endowment, available subsidies, and the formula of division of costs. Relationships may be benign or bitter, depending upon personalities and the financial situation of each party. Conflicts heated up as third-party payments from Blue Cross and then from government agencies began to be made on a per-diem cost basis, and as HMOs and other comprehensive prepayment organizations saw marked differences between teaching hospitals and community hospitals in cost for the same diagnosis and treatment. These financial relationships are now of major importance as a pro-competition philosophy and the prospective pricing system utilizing DRGs are being implemented by the federal government as the new strategy for containment of Medicare costs.

In the early 1940s the answer seemed very simple. Patient care in teaching hospitals cost 15 percent more than in large, nonteaching hospitals. This ratio became almost an axiom, and I blush now as I recall its origin. Basil MacLean was asked to consult with the New York Hospital–Cornell Medical School complex in New York City on financial relationships, and I accompanied him. One of our tasks was to compare the published per-diem costs of the major teaching hospitals in New York City (New York Hospital and Columbia-Presbyterian) with those of other large hospitals, such as Mt. Sinai, St. Luke's, Lenox Hill, and Roosevelt. The teaching hospitals' costs turned out to be at least 15 percent higher. Without any further analysis we concluded that the 15 percent discrepancy was due to the added costs associated with a university teaching hospital. The figure was accepted uncritically for a number of years. (This was the same type of unscientific reasoning that led to the acceptance of 4.5 hospital beds per 1,000 population as a norm for the country as a whole—with 3.0 beds per 1,000 needed in rural areas and 6.0 beds per 1,000 in larger referral or metropolitan areas.)

Basil MacLean and I took for granted that the costs associated with the teaching hospital were greater, but we believed that we were running our institution prudently and that the additional cost was justified. Our center was well-endowed, and both the hospital and the medical school were owned by the university. As I have related, the situation in New Haven—an independent university teaching hospital with only a small endowment and dependent upon a large annual cash subsidy from the university—was very different. Because I was fighting for the hospital's fiscal survival in New Haven, I made every effort to keep costs down. I reviewed every budget of every department with the director of personnel, the controller and the assistant director, as well as with the department heads. I opposed increases in personnel and was niggardly in wage scales and chintzy in capital expenditures. When I presented the budget and suggested rates for the coming year to the board, I was always confident that it was as lean as it could be and I was prepared to defend it to anyone.

I had no doubt, however, that the presence of the medical school increased hospital costs. The reasons became clear when I took the department heads to visit Frank Sutton at the Miami Valley Hospital in Dayton, Ohio, to compare operating costs. That hospital was quite comparable to Grace-New Haven in patient census, capacity, and types of services provided—but its overall costs were substantially lower. Our unit costs for dietary, nursing, business office, and administrative activities were quite close. Radiology and pathology were also not very far apart— although more tests were ordered in the university hospital, the additional costs were offset by the salaried arrangements in New Haven. But New Haven's maintenance, housekeeping, and utilities costs, as well as the costs of some special services, such as the operating room, were substantially higher. The greater amount of space required for the university hospital's educational activities accounted for the first three items. The operating room cost more because many operations took longer. Our analyses showed that the operating room of a teaching hospital was on the average occupied thirty minutes longer than if a private patient were being operated upon by an experienced surgeon. The new surgeon or resident obviously cannot function as rapidly as an experienced one, and the same applies to the anesthesiology resident. This did not affect the quality of care: the professor or senior resident was always present at the operation, functioning as either chief surgeon or first assistant and keeping the younger doctor under direct observation. But it was inevitable that the resident would work more slowly. It is thus both natural and proper that a teaching hospital will use more personnel and space in the operating room or in other areas concerned with teaching.

Probably the biggest difference between Miami Valley and New Haven was in patient mix and services to ambulatory patients. The Ohio hospital had a relatively low percentage of nonpaying patients, while in New Haven over 50 percent of the patients could not pay the full hospital charges. Thus bad debts and free service were an appreciable part of our costs, and they were substantially lower in Miami Valley. Of even greater significance to our deficit were ambulatory services, which were provided at low or no cost to low-income residents of the New Haven area. Not only were patients usually unable to pay for the visit, medicines, and special services, but a larger amount of space was required to see them. A private doctor can see ten to forty patients a day in a few consulting and examining rooms. A teaching outpatient department, on the other hand, requires examination and treatment areas for the medical students, and each visit takes substantially longer because the student has to work up the patient and then bring in the attending physician, who also reviews and examines the patient. Finally, the two discuss diagnosis and treatment. The necessity for consultation makes the educational process more time-costly than private examinations.

As more accurate and detailed cost analyses were developed in the late 1940s and early 1950s, we could identify other areas in which teaching hospitals had legitimately higher costs. For one, teaching patients undergo more examinations—sometimes because their condition requires them, but more often because the student or resident must be certain that everything possible has been done in anticipation of teaching rounds with the attending physician. I still recall my pleasure as an intern and resident when the professor would suggest some esoteric test, and I was able modestly to describe the results. I can also recall the times when the attending physician gently implied that only a muddle-headed practitioner would neglect to carry out a certain procedure I had forgotten. For years, the administration tried without success to inculcate cost concern into the attending and teaching staffs. Medical schools and teaching hospitals are now making greater efforts to emphasize the importance of costs in health care. But governmental, industrial, and other third-party payers must also recognize that in a teaching institution the students and resident staff must be exposed to the latest developments and procedures.

Length of Stay

Teaching hospitals have been accused of keeping patients in the hospital longer than necessary. This was once a legitimate criticism, but it is substantially less true today. At New Haven, I compared the length of our patients' stays with the figures published periodically by the United Hospital Fund of New York. As a rule, patients stayed at Grace-New Haven for shorter periods of time. Although I would love to credit the difference to the ability of the hospital administrator or the cost-consciousness of the faculty and attending physicians, I suspect the primary reason was the relative shortage of hospital beds in New Haven. This shortage meant there was a waiting list in the teaching component of Grace-New Haven. Each resident stopped every day at the admitting office with his or her list of patients to be admitted and reviewed with the admitting officer and the nurses on the floor the patients who could safely be discharged.

On the other hand, many other cities have too many hospital beds. Whatever the other advantages or disadvantages of the DRGs, this program and the high cost of hospital care have prompted a much more critical look at the number of acute care hospital beds in each community or region, with the conclusion that many areas have too many beds. A number of hospitals are reducing capacity or even closing. This problem is not only applicable to teaching hospitals but is a major factor in the efficient utilization of expensive facilities in all hospitals. Milton Roemer of UCLA has the dubious distinction of having identified Roemer's Law, which essentially states that any empty hospital bed will soon be occupied. The process also works in reverse; in New Haven, the shortage of hospital beds helped keep hospital stays down. Competent, professional health facility planning for an area, a region, or a state is the best way to provide the highest quality health care for that region. This is why I encouraged close cooperation between the university teaching hospital, the associated community and neighboring hospitals, and ambulatory and long-term care facilities in developing patterns to provide for a continuum of care. I felt that the major university teaching hospitals should assume leadership in this regard, not only because they should work cooperatively with their associates, but because they are especially vulnerable to criticism, with their higher costs and their occasional difficulties in discharging patients when medically indicated. (This is partly due to their higher percentage of poor patients, those who have precarious family situations, and those who have long, complicated illnesses, such as the elderly.)

FINANCIAL ENTANGLEMENTS

For many years, Grace-New Haven reduced costs by employing salaried hospital-based specialists and by charging professional fees to hospitalized clinic patients who happened to have medical insurance through their employment but who could not afford private physicians otherwise. The income was used to offset the cost of the resident staff. As I discussed in chapter 5, the hospital-based specialists on salary retained their professional independence; their incomes were comparable to those in clinical specialties; but they still provided service at a lower cost. The senior resident staff charged professional fees to medically indigent clinic patients who, through employment, had commercial insurance or Blue Shield for professional fees. The fees were billed through the medical school's Office of Professional Services and then turned over to the hospital, which paid the resident staff's salaries and expenses. We were careful to report this offsetting income in our calculations for cost reimbursement to Blue Cross and Medicare.

Substantial changes have occurred since Medicare was enacted in 1965. In a number of teaching hospitals, including Yale-New Haven, surgical pathology, anesthesiology, and radiology have shifted from the hospital to the medical school, or to a private operation. Today, Yale-New Haven is still responsible for the salaries and expenses of the resident

staff, but most of the professional fees for clinic patients or from Medicare
are collected and kept by the Medical School, which has assumed more
direct responsibility in order to comply with Medicare requirements. The
resident staff is now essentially a direct cost to the hospital which brings
in relatively little offsetting income.

As financial relationships between hospital and medical school
change, continued attention must be paid to charging practices and costs
for both partners. The public must be made to understand and support
the justifiably higher costs of these unique institutions. But on the other
hand, the medical centers and hospitals must be prepared to demonstrate
that they are not taking financial advantage of their unique position. This
will not be easy, for the world of medical education is beset with financial
problems that seem to be increasing in size and complexity. These issues
are not new; they have simply been exacerbated by external pressures.

I became concerned with the separation of costs between medical
school and university teaching hospitals in my first year at Strong Memorial Hospital. The University of Rochester had a contract with the city by
which it ran the Rochester Municipal Hospital patient divisions as an
operating unit of SMH. The costs of all services, from nursing to maintenance to dietary, were prorated on the basis of the number of patient days
in either of the two hospitals. This meant, first, that all patients received
the same quality and amount of service—but it also meant that the costs
of teaching and research in the medical center, which could not be
justified as directly related to patient service, had to be eliminated from
the hospital's bill to the city. The contract contained a clause that many
people found laughable because it seemed so unlegalistic:

The parties hereto recognize the fact that the relation between the medical school
and the hospital of the University and the Municipal Hospital will necessarily be
intimate and interdependent and that each will derive the greatest benefit only by
promoting the interest of both and each of the parties hereto is, therefore, entering
into the contract with the intention of loyally cooperating with the other in
carrying out the terms of the contract and agrees to interpret its provisions, insofar
as it may legally do so, in such a manner as will best promote the interests of both
and render the highest service to the public.

Basil MacLean and I considered this clause as important as all of the
preceding twenty-five. It expressed the philosophy that I brought to New
Haven and it was essentially the basis upon which Drs. Darling, Blake,
and Long and I worked on the first major revision of the agreement
between Grace-New Haven Hospital and Yale University.

By the late 1940s and early 1950s, cost accounting and cost analyses
had become more sophisticated, and the accepted common chart of

accounts enabled much more accurate comparisons to be made. Hospital per-diem costs had also mounted rapidly after the war. I had helped develop both the Connecticut statute that required the state or town to pay the actual costs of hospital care for state welfare patients and the AHA principles of reimbursement, and I had become very aware of the high per-diem costs at Grace-New Haven—for a number of years, they were the highest in the state. An obvious question was whether these hospital expenses included teaching and research costs that should properly be borne by the medical school and the university. Since in the late 1940s and early 1950s we had to assume radiology and laboratory costs that had previously been financed by the medical school, I was not eager to reopen this issue. I knew that my per-diem costs were high and I tried each year to cut. But I also knew that the institution was unique in Connecticut in the depth and variety of service it offered, and this fact was not unrelated to its intimate association with a medical school.

As I became more active in the AHA and in the teaching hospital section of the AAMC, I became more interested in the financial relationships between teaching hospitals and medical schools. To my delight, Ward Darley and Augustus Carroll of the AAMC agreed to undertake a major study of the subject. Gus drew up the preliminary protocol with input from Darley, Dean Vernon Lippard of the Yale Medical School, and me. The Yale Medical School and Grace-New Haven were used for the trial run.

The preliminary pilot study took forever to complete. We found, to our collective embarrassment, that Yale's was one of the few medical schools that had never had an AAMC financial study. A rough draft of the report was finally sent to me for comment just as I was leaving for Japan to visit the Atomic Bomb Casualty Commission. I wrote my comments to Ward Darley on a rainy afternoon in Nagasaki. When I returned, Dr. Darley asked if the letter could be incorporated in the final report. I was flattered, particularly as Gus Carroll had recently died and the expanded AAMC had subjected his work to a far more sophisticated analysis.[4]

My comments, written in 1968, reflected my conviction that the medical school and the hospital must understand and share equitably the expenses of their medical center. I was also aware, even at that early date, of the growing concern of third-party payers over steadily increasing costs and the need to assure them that they were paying for an identifiable product. Dr. Darley added in a footnote in the final manuscript that he agreed and went on to say, "If the study shows that the present house staff

4. A. J. Carroll, "Program Cost Estimating in a Teaching Hospital," Thomas J. Campbell and Mary H. Lillemeyer, eds., Association of American Medical Colleges, 1969.

situation is one that requires a study that can lead to the establishment of long-needed, long-range policies, I believe that this in itself justifies the publication of this report."

Basil MacLean's and my original estimate that teaching hospitals' costs are at least 15 percent higher than those of nonteaching hospitals is probably as accurate as any yet presented. It is to the credit of those who create the DRG reimbursement formulae that this extra cost is taken into consideration. But administrators of teaching hospitals are concerned that, as Medicare costs continue to rise and funds are less available, this added reimbursement will probably be cut away. The burden of assuring fair reimbursement falls equally upon the teaching hospital, the medical school, and the individual or third-party payer. The teaching hospital must recognize that its expenses and services are not automatically acceptable merely because it is associated with medical education—it must assure that its operations are efficient and its services of the highest quality. The medical school, in turn, must not expect the teaching hospital or the paying patient to make up for decreasing grants or educational deficits. At the same time, the payer and the public must recognize the important contribution that teaching hospitals make to health care. No payment formula should ignore any of the four responsibilities of the teaching hospital: teaching, research, patient care, and community service.

THE TEACHING HOSPITAL AND THE COMMUNITY

The community responsibilities of the university teaching hospital were not high on my priority list in my early days of hospital administration. My early publications concerned standard insurance forms, decentralized refrigeration, improved sterilization in the utility rooms, and various mechanisms for economy of operation, reflecting my primary interests in the administration and internal operation of the hospital. But Basil MacLean's activities in Blue Cross and state and national hospital associations and my increased responsibilities in New Haven forced me to extend my sight beyond the hospital building. Increased involvement in state and national hospital affairs also stimulated this broader concern.

My responsibilities as a hospital executive required my active participation in the community, but at least two additional influences increased my involvement. One was the development of outpatient services in other hospitals similar to mine. These included the remarkable homecare program initiated by E. M. Bluestone out of Montefiore Hospital in New York City; the program of the Bingham Associates from the Tufts Medical Center, which supported pathologists and radiologists in hospitals in northern New England; the Pratt Diagnostic Center and the Columbia Point Project in an underserved section of Boston; MGH's efforts in another outlying section of Boston; the group practice developed by George Baehr at Mt. Sinai in New York City and his battles with leaders of organized medicine, who were fighting group practice by imposing sanctions on hospital privileges; and the attempts of Johns Hopkins to improve health care in its immediate neighborhood as well as its exciting excursion into a complete medical care program in Columbia, Maryland. I was also impressed with the activity of the Michael Reese Hospital in Chicago, which obviously had a profound effect on the neighborhood and community around it. All these successful programs made me feel that my own institution could and should provide greater service to the community than merely caring for patients in its emergency room, clinics, and beds.

My other stimulus came out of my own "milkmaid's stool" speech to the AAMC in 1959, in which I had enumerated the three responsibilities of the teaching hospital as teaching, research, and patient care. The reactions I received from my academic colleagues, the work of other institutions, and my long-range planning for my own medical center combined to add a fourth leg to my institutional stool—community service. I discussed my growing conviction in a speech to the New England Hospital Assembly in the early 1960s. The hospital maintenance department made me a small three-legged stool and a four-legged stool, each with one detachable leg. For each stool they also made a slightly shorter leg. In the speech I showed that the three-legged stool could stand solidly even with one short leg—but the four-legged stool was clearly unsteady if all legs were not the same. I was trying to point out the greater difficulty of assuming all four responsibilities, but I also hoped to convince my audience that all four were important and that an effort should be made to keep them in balance. I also had a one-hundred-dollar bill pinned to the easel to illustrate my prediction that daily hospital costs were inevitably going to rise to this level and beyond. They laughed at me, and I may have spoiled my goal of selling community service with my seemingly outrageous cost prediction. A few years later, MGH's John Knowles drew similar hoots with a thousand-dollar-a-day prediction.

I continue to have the uncomfortable feeling that the teaching hospital, this vital component of the health world, is unduly vulnerable because its unavoidably higher costs stand out. The medical centers must be preserved and supported so that their contributions can continue. This requires the understanding of local communities, states, and community health organizations. This is why I emphasized the importance of the fourth leg of the stool—community service. Not only should the medical students and resident staff be exposed to their future responsibilities and relations with the local community and its health agencies, but the medical center itself should work in collaboration—not in competition—with these health partners.[5]

This presents an interesting challenge to the administration and board of the teaching hospital. Not only should there be strong horizontal collaboration with other teaching hospitals through COTH or such recently formed organizations as the Federation of Voluntary Hospitals, but local patient care corporations, consortia, or collaborations should also be seriously considered. The teaching hospital should take the initiative in helping plan to provide for a continuum of care in the local community.

If all this sounds as if I am wistfully recalling the good old days, I submit that the atmosphere today seems unnecessarily uncooperative, suspicious, and competitive. With these attitudes comes the danger that the care of the patient as a person will no longer be the primary objective of the hospital, its administration, and its staff. I regard with considerable misgivings the efforts of prominent teaching hospitals to develop a second- or third-tier corporate structure (discussed in chapter 7) and to involve profit-making enterprises. Home health care is an example of a service that may suffer from such activities. Third-party payers are pushing for earlier discharge and more home health care and long-term care institutions. But local nonprofit home health care agencies that have existed for years may be bypassed in favor of commercial agencies, perhaps set up as loss leaders in order to sell more profitable services, such as drugs and medical supplies. Any program that offers two levels of care—for those who can and cannot pay—is in the long run deleterious to both the community and the medical center. On the other hand, the hospital that becomes involved in home care and long-term care can enhance the total program of care in the community. Of course, it is the responsibility of the community to finance health care for those who cannot afford it.

HEALTH CARE FOR LOW-INCOME PATIENTS

One of the teaching hospital's major community contributions, by circumstance or tradition, is the provision of health care for patients who

5. A. S. Relman reinforces this responsibility of the teaching hospitals to the community and public in his thoughtful article "Who Will Pay for Medical Education in our Teaching Hospitals?" (*Science* 226, October 1984, pp. 20–23). I can only add that this pertains to all teaching hospitals—not just the 115 institutions discussed in such detail in the report of the Task Force on Academic Health Centers (*Prescription for Change*, Commonwealth Fund, 1985).

cannot pay. At first, these patients were considered teaching material, but when I entered hospital administration in Rochester and in New Haven, all patients received the basic professional and support services regardless of the source—or lack—of funds to pay for their care. When a patient came to the emergency room, he or she was treated and, if necessary, admitted. We didn't require payment in advance or turn patients away because they were in financial need.

This attitude was not particularly businesslike by any criteria I know of—but it was the philosophy of many hospitals, and I took it for granted. I have already related my early efforts to get the government to assume complete financial responsibility for welfare patients, poor mothers and children, veterans' dependents, and, later, Medicare and Medicaid recipients. It took me longer to understand the problem of the medically indigent or working poor. These were families or individuals who were self-supporting under normal circumstances but unable to meet the extraordinary expenses of a serious illness—especially if the patient was the family wage earner. As the costs of health care increased, these cases mounted. Unless the hospital reimbursement formula provided for free or reduced-charge care and bad debts, or overcharged paying patients, subsidizing the medically indigent became a very important factor in the hospital's fiscal stability.

This problem was particularly serious at Yale-New Haven and in the other hospital in New Haven, St. Raphael. Sister Louise, its CEO, and I jointly publicized the problem of financing health care for the medically indigent. As a result, the state welfare commissioner, Bernard Shapiro, who was remarkable in his understanding of people's needs, established a blue-ribbon commission under the leadership of a well-known public utility executive. The commission's findings were carefully reviewed by the local mayors, first selectmen, and welfare officers. Common understandings and policies were developed among the cities and towns, and the state welfare department, so that all shared in the cost of underwriting a portion of the expense.

This occurred in the early 1960s, before Medicare and Medicaid, and before the question was raised as to whether health care was a right or a privilege. In retrospect, it is clear that I believed health care was a right (I still do), and that hospitals, professionals, and the community were obliged to provide such care. But who should pay for it? I felt it was a responsibility of society, and that the teaching hospital should make whatever contribution it could in skills and services. In those days, it was not suggested that such problems could be solved through competition. My guess is that, if someone had suggested such an approach for providing health services and controlling rising costs, my response would have been, "how does one mount a successful, competitive program for patients who cannot pay?"

Throughout my career, I have been impressed by the high-quality health care that teaching hospitals have given to those who could not pay—particularly by the resident staff, the cost of whose education worries so many.[6] I am also well aware of the massive problems of public hospitals that are almost exclusively for the poor. These are the institutions of last resort, to whom other hospitals transfer (the polite word for "dump") patients who cannot pay, or who are not socially or professionally acceptable. These hospitals, along with many small, rural hospitals, and teaching hospitals, carry a disproportionate share of medically indigent patients, those who are not eligible for welfare but who cannot afford health care.

In 1946, I could not collect on the full cost of the services the hospital provided in approximately 50 percent of the cases. Neither Grace-New Haven nor the Yale Medical School could have survived if we had not been able to obtain fair reimbursement from the government for indigent patients. The same situation applies today, particularly in hospitals located in large, low-income areas, or when competition shifts the patient population so that a greater proportion of indigent patients are admitted to the teaching hospital. This is not a problem that can be solved by an improved economy of operation. The states and the federal government must pay for the health care of those unable to pay for it themselves, just as medical schools and teaching hospitals must accept their responsibility for providing high quality care at the lowest cost possible.

I can only repeat that the great teaching hospitals—or health centers, as they like to be termed—must deserve this support on the basis of the contribution they make, and their willingness to collaborate in deeds, not talk. I am well aware of medical schools' need for funds for medical education and research. But undue profits from hospital specialties in either medical schools or hospitals, as well as from commercial pharmacies and home health care programs set up at the expense of the long-standing community agencies, may erode the support these academic health centers must continue to have. The first to suffer if this support wanes will be the indigent and medically indigent patients.

Although I emphasize the role and the responsibility of the teaching hospitals in caring for the indigent, I would be remiss if I did not recognize

6. The report of the Task Force on Academic Health Centers (*Prescription for Change*) states, "teaching hospitals, in the aggregate, constitute less than 6% of the nation's acute care hospitals, but they provide more than 47% of the nation's free medical care."

the major contributions to this type of care by all types of hospitals as well as by many physicians. I appreciated the statements of concern by Thomas Matherlee and Alexander McMahon of the AHA, and I also applaud the comments of Scott Parker, who became chairman of the Board of Trustees of the AHA in 1986. He correctly assessed the magnitude of the problem of caring for the uninsured, the poor, and the aged, and he challenged all components of our society to share in this responsibility— voluntary and proprietary health systems of all types and government at all levels. They must collectively face the challenge to improve efficiency in the delivery of care and must assure equitable distribution of the expense. But society must set the policy of providing health care for all people.

POST-GRADUATE MEDICAL EDUCATION

The resident staff, in a hospital of sufficient size and quality to support it, is a unique element in our health care system, an intimate part of the hospital's medical staff that plays a vital role in providing medical services to hospital patients and to the community. I have been fortunate in that the three university teaching hospitals with which I have been associated all had superb internship and residency programs. I always felt that the resident staff and the nurses were the most critical judges of the ability of the attending medical staff and the care they provided. I had more confidence in their evaluations of physicians and hospital operations than in most academic criteria or indices. Admittedly their evaluations are subjective, and I may be making too much of my personal experiences. But when I was on the resident staff at Stanford and the pediatric staff at Rochester, my colleagues and I quickly learned which physicians were competent, conscientious and concerned with the welfare of the patient, and which were mediocre. We knew which ones we would want to take care of us or our families.

I regarded the resident staff so highly that a few years after I came to Grace-New Haven I formed an unofficial junior medical board made up of senior residents. Their merciless evaluations of the inadequacies of the administration, the nurses, and the medical staff were invaluable to me. But it was hard to get them to stop talking about remaking the institution or my administrative organization!

A critical and independent group of young physicians who are on the front lines in the care of patients is one of the greatest assets a hospital administrator can have. It is not easy to work with them, however, for they are still learning—but often don't believe it. An excellent example of this attitude is the "LMD (local medical doctor) syndrome." The interns and residents are usually the first to see patients on admission. Most of the private patients have their own doctors. Unlike the vast majority of these doctors' patients, they did not get well and reached a stage where hospitalization was needed. The resident staff thus sees the patient when symptoms have advanced, and a battery of sophisticated tests and examinations are easily available to them. As a result, definitive diagnoses frequently become evident following admission. The resident staff then wonders why the LMD was so ignorant as not to have seen the problem. As the wisecrack goes, the resident's definition of a healthy patient is one who has not yet been completely worked up.

Unfortunately, the resident staff's attitude of superiority is sometimes encouraged by medical school faculty, who are eager to enhance the reputation of their service. In many teaching hospitals, private physicians are expected to give their orders through the resident staff. Sometimes they find that their orders have been delayed or countermanded. This interference has occasionally resulted in serious breaches between attending physicians and teaching institutions. I was fortunate in this regard—in New Haven, I could review the attitudes of the resident staff, private patients, and their community physicians with the community chief of service and the university chief, so that a relatively even balance could be preserved. There is really little question as to what is fair and proper. The patient selects and depends on a physician, and he or she must have final responsibility for that patient in the hospital. There must be a compelling reason before any other physician, senior or resident, interferes.

I always believed that most community physicians appreciated the resident staff's care of their patients, partly because they stimulated the older doctors to keep up to date, but also because they eased demands on their time, particularly at night and in emergencies. Sometimes, however, their pocketbooks spoke more loudly than their professional pride, to the extent that community physicians occasionally discouraged senior residents from establishing practice in the community. (Faculty were occasionally guilty of this as well.) One chief at SMH would not appoint a new resident unless he or she agreed not to go into practice within one hundred miles of Rochester after finishing his or her residency. This requirement apparently had been accepted without question for a number of years before Dr. MacLean and I heard of it, when one particularly competent resident and his wife wanted to stay in Rochester. We didn't bother to find out whether the original agreement was legal—we just raised hell with the chief of service and forced him to withdraw the restriction.

Another specialty chief refused to allow two of his residents to lease his clinical practice facilities in the medical center, even though he was not using the facilities. Another resident, a superb clinician with over six years' specialty training in the hospital, needed to borrow two thousand dollars to tide him over his first few months in practice. These problems had simple solutions. In return for supervising the hospital clinic in which they had trained, I allowed them to use hospital space and staff for their private patients until they had built up a profitable practice. I also called the bank president, who was also president of the hospital board, and told him I would guarantee the resident's loan. He agreed on one condition: he had to share in the guarantee. All three physicians were out on their own within six months and all are among the most respected practitioners in the community.

I suppose the resident staff would say that I appreciated their contributions and supported them more because I was so niggardly with their stipends. For years, they complained that MGH, Johns Hopkins Hospital, Lakeside Hospital in Cleveland, Barnes Hospital in St. Louis, and Grace-New Haven were competing to pay the lowest salary. They might be correct. Grace-New Haven, however, was one of the first hospitals to convert benefits into salary so that the increasing number of married residents could live with their families. We also led the way in covering them with malpractice insurance. Edwin Crosby of Hopkins and I first pressed for a nationwide internship matching plan, which the AAMC began work on in 1949–1950. When Dr. Crosby moved from Johns Hopkins to the JCAH and then to the AHA, this program was refined. A formal program became a practical necessity as competition among hospitals for interns intensified, and juniors in medical school were being pressed into commitments almost twenty months before graduation. Medical schools, hospitals, and chiefs of service were developing an unseemly practice of undercover negotiations and commitments that were unfair to all—particularly the medical students. The National Resident Matching Program (NRMP) turned out to be an important contribution to both medical students and hospitals. But John A. D. Cooper, president of the AAMC, reported in 1983 and 1984 that residency program directors in several specialties were beginning to adopt early timetables and selection processes incompatible with the NRMP.[7] Presumably more education and negotiation are needed.

When we started paying the resident staff decent wages, my conscience was never bothered when I battled with the third-party payment

7. J. A. D. Cooper, "AAMC President's Weekly Activity Report," May 26, 1983; December 6, 1984.

agencies for inclusion of their salaries as a legitimate part of hospital costs. Grace-New Haven was the locus of the first detailed study of the time interns and residents spent caring for patients in the hospital. I could not believe the figures reported by Henry Payson in his 1961 study,[8] so another study was done in which a medical student essentially lived with an intern or resident for a week. Some residents were on service 110–120 hours per week, and the entire staff averaged more than 70 hours per week. These studies left little doubt in my mind that residents were providing at least 40 hours or more of service alone, and that their additional hours were both education and service. I even concluded that their work week was not substantially less than mine had been in 1932–37—even though I never admitted this publicly.

Resident staff's salaries have risen markedly over the past decade and are clearly a factor in the increased cost of teaching hospitals today. Sensitive as I am to the cost of health care, I was never disturbed by the cost of the resident staff—particularly when we were able to apply their professional earnings to hospital costs. We also began to challenge some specialty boards' requirements for extra years of training in the basic sciences or an additional year of residency—which came at the hospital's or the patients' expense. Another factor should be considered in justifying residents' salaries. The four years of medical school education are four years of great expense and little or no income. The majority of medical students incur debts and forgo the earnings of their college classmates who did not elect four more years of graduate school, plus one to six years residency training.

Government agencies, particularly the Health Care Financing Administration, Blue Cross and Blue Shield, commercial insurance companies, and the public are to be congratulated for recognizing that postgraduate medical education is a legitimate cost in teaching hospitals. This support must continue, and medical schools and teaching hospitals, through AAMC, COTH, the AMA, the AHA, and the specialty societies, must continue to justify and monitor these programs. They must be prepared to take steps to limit both overproduction of doctors, particularly graduates of foreign medical schools, and specialty groups' efforts to increase required years of training.

I can offer from personal experience and observation, both as an intern and resident and later as an administrator, my admiration for these young physicians and my conviction that their advanced training is of

8. H. E. Payson, E. C. Gaenslen, Jr., F. L. Stargardter, "Time Study of an Internship on a University Medical Service," *New England Journal of Medicine* 264, 9 (1961), 439–43.

value. The professional service the resident staff provides to indigent patients, for which no professional fee is available, is irreplaceable. I have seen them in action in emergency situations in the hospital and have seen them develop into excellent physicians, and I strongly advocate that their training be supported.

7

The Health Care System

The preceding chapters have partly described the evolution from a doctor trained to diagnose and treat a patient's illness to a doctor concerned with his or her patients' overall health and welfare and, beyond that, with the health of the environment itself—neighbors and community. The emphasis of the earlier doctor's training was on the patient in an acute-care institution. Other aspects of the system that provided people with health and sickness care were ignored, as was how a patient obtained health care or paid for it. It was not until I started working with Basil MacLean in hospital administration that I was introduced to problems of sick people as a group, as contrasted to those of individuals. I then began to appreciate the enormity and complexity of this country's health system, the many components that were so inextricably mixed that they had to be considered, not only for their own importance, but because of their impact upon each other.

PUBLIC HEALTH

In the spring of my residency year, I was invited to become the deputy health officer in Olean, Cattaraugus county, in western New York. My wife and I were impressed with the staff and intrigued by their offer to finance us for advanced degrees in public health at Johns Hopkins after a year or so at Olean. But we arrived on the wrong day. A diagnosis of diphtheria had just been made in an adjoining community, and our interviews were continually interrupted by reports and discussions on the condition of the sick child. His attending physician was giving him what seemed to me and to the public health staff virtually homeopathic doses of antitoxin. The protracted arguments were not over the appropriate dose, however, but how best to persuade the attending physician to give adequate medication. After listening to this soul-searching for several hours, I could keep quiet no longer. "Why don't you tell the doctor he is not treating the patient properly, and if necessary, get one of his local colleagues who knows the proper treatment to talk with you both?" Their response was very plain: public health officials do not interfere with the health care of individual patients. Their treatment is the sole prerogative of the attending physician. My wife and I thanked our hosts for their hospitality, returned to Rochester, and politely declined the appointment. I did not think I could last long in that type of environment, and I began to appreciate more the stories that William Snow and my father-in-law, Thomas Storey, had told me of their experiences in the American Social Hygiene Association which worked to prevent and treat venereal disease among the troops during the two world wars. Many local physicians indignantly refused or rejected their suggestions to test the patients' contacts, calling the social hygienists "public health interferers."

I was reminded of both these incidents when I went to Illinois in 1969 as coordinator of health services. The board of the Illinois Medical Society graciously invited my wife and me to dinner and spent most of the evening telling us about their very clear understanding with the director of health that medical and health care were the prerogative of the practicing physicians, not government or public health officials.

Courses in public health, which might have broadened the vision of young physicians, were relatively unimportant in the curriculum of Stanford Medical School in the 1930s. Likewise, the University of Rochester School of Medicine did not even have a division of public health, and interest in community health and community medicine did not come to this school until many years later. So my public health horizons were broadened markedly when, on coming to New Haven in 1946, I met C. E. A. Winslow and Ira Hiscock, the first and second chairmen of the Department of Public Health in the Yale Medical School. From them I learned not only that nutrition, housing and environment were important health factors but also that medical care was considered a respected function of the Department of Public Health. Franz Goldman, Milton Roemer, and Jonas Muller were pioneers in this field, followed by my own recruits, Falk and Weinerman. Not until Arthur Viseltear described in 1973 the development of the medical care section of the American Public Health Association (APHA) in 1948 did I realize how bitterly even sincere and respected members of the public health community, such as Haven Emerson of Columbia, fought its formation.[1] I had never fully recognized how strong

1. A. J. Viseltear, "Emergency of the Medical Care Section of the APHA, 1926–1948: A Chapter in the History of Medical Care," *AJPH* 63 (1973), 986–1007.

and widespread was the feeling that public health officials should do nothing that might be construed as interfering with medical care by physicians. It also became clear to me that, while this attitude was fostered by physicians and organized medicine, many public health officials themselves hesitated to extend their field of responsibility.

VOLUNTARY HEALTH INSURANCE

The first component of the overall health system that I became aware of as a budding hospital administrator was voluntary health insurance for hospital charges, and then for physicians' fees. Dr. MacLean had been one of the pioneers in this field, having helped develop both a local Blue Cross program, in New Orleans, and a national one. He believed that nonprofit health insurance was crucial in preserving the financial resources of the voluntary health system. I think this is true. It is interesting to speculate on what the position of the British voluntary hospitals would have been after World War II if there had been a strong Blue Cross system in that nation.

Having learned from Dr. MacLean of the contributions of Blue Cross and having seen that all segments of the community, including the local county medical society, gave their support to the highly regarded Rochester plan, I took it for granted that Blue Cross had been enthusiastically welcomed throughout the country. I soon had a rude awakening. I was sitting between Dr. MacLean and Robin Buerki in a large auditorium in Chicago in the early 1940s, listening to Morris Fishbein, editor of the AMA Journal, speak on national health from the point of view of the AMA. When he started praising Blue Cross and emphasizing the AMA's wholehearted support, I was suddenly almost crushed by two large men leaning toward each other across me. Loudly and indignantly they recalled that the AMA and its spokesman—the same Dr. Fishbein—had fought tooth and nail against Blue Cross, calling it "half-baked, socialized medicine." The AHA had been the primary supporter and promoter of voluntary prepayment Blue Cross from the early 1930s, and these two administrators had been among those in the hospital world who encouraged its support and expansion over bitter AMA opposition.

I began to understand the view of organized medicine that Blue Cross represented "socialism" when two of my neighbors in Rochester joined the local doctors in trying to educate me. They represented commercial insurance companies and were finding it very difficult to sell their highly publicized and theoretically cheaper hospital insurance policies in the community. They were particularly indignant that most of the major industries in Rochester—particularly Eastman Kodak—supported the local Blue Cross program of "community" ratings for premiums rather than "experience" ratings for individual companies. Many Blue Cross plans had across-the-board community ratings in the late 1930s and 1940s. By supporting these, larger companies could indirectly subsidize the overall health costs of the community.

The community ratings philosophy was embraced by many leaders in the hospital and nonprofit health insurance industry. It was admittedly somewhat idealistic, but it was strengthened by the genuine partnership of hospitals and Blue Cross at the local and national levels, a relationship rewarding to both sides. Connecticut Blue Cross (CBC) was also interested in such a partnership. When I discovered that the Philadelphia Blue Cross plan contributed financially to the Philadelphia Hospital Council, I approached CBC about similar financial support for the newly reorganizing Connecticut Hospital Association (CHA). They received five to ten thousand dollars annually from CBC for a number of years, until the new organization became strongly established. Later, when CBC had financial difficulties, the Connecticut hospitals agreed to a limited moratorium of payments from CBC for a number of months, while it reorganized its premium and benefit schedules. The CBC subsequently repaid the hospitals with interest.

Community rating gradually disappeared as competition with commercial companies using experience rating increased. Competition was encouraged during World War II, when the Wage Stabilization Board ruled that the provision of hospital benefits under new contract settlements did not violate the National Wage Stabilization Act. The later ruling that such benefits qualified as legitimate business expenses for employers, and did not constitute reportable income for employees increased the pressure to provide them.

The Blue Cross movement, once housed in two small offices at AHA headquarters, grew into a major nonprofit program, with a continuing close partnership with hospitals. It expanded from a commission in the AHA structure into a national body, the Blue Cross Association. Basil MacLean became its first president in 1956. His influence preserved the close relationship between Blue Cross and the hospitals, which continued during a brief period of interim leadership by another Blue Cross pioneer, James E. B. Stuart, and Walter J. McNerney's presidency, beginning in 1962. This partnership was beneficial to both the public and the health care providers. The working relationship between the AHA and Blue Cross was nationally significant during the years leading up to the passage of Medicare in 1965 and during its subsequent implementation. After the development of Medicare rules, regulations and guidelines, the next national problem was the selection of intermediaries for the government in various parts of the country. Blue Cross and commercial insurance companies both wanted the privilege, and in many areas the hospital's preference for Blue Cross as their Part A (hospital costs) intermediary was accepted by the Department of Social Security within Health, Education, and Welfare (HEW).

When the time came to select a Medicare intermediary, Connecticut found itself in an unusual situation. Home for several of the largest and best commercial insurance companies, Connecticut also had a fine Blue Cross plan. The CHA was designated to transmit to HEW the opinions of the Connecticut hospitals regarding the intermediary. The AHA had strongly endorsed Blue Cross. The executive director of the Hartford Hospital, T. Stewart Hamilton, had been president of the AHA in 1963 and had worked with the AHA on the Medicare legislation. But many of the members of Dr. Hamilton's board of directors and of the boards of the other hospitals in the Hartford area were associated with the Hartford insurance companies. While Dr. Hamilton was in Chicago planning the AHA strategy on Medicare intermediaries, the Hartford area boards met and chose commercial insurance intermediaries. The local hospitals were divided between Aetna and Travelers for Part A and all supported Connecticut General for Medicare Part B (medical services). Dr. Hamilton returned to a fait accompli, and I suspect that he heaved a sigh of relief.

I favored Blue Cross for Part A, but I knew the hospitals had to make their own decisions. The CHA met one morning with representatives of Blue Cross and that afternoon with the Hartford insurance companies. Stewart Hamilton did a masterful job of explaining the AHA position as well as the decision of the Hartford group of hospitals. I found myself taking on the role of primary inquisitor in both sessions. No doubt my prejudices were evident. The CHA finally recommended Blue Cross as the Part A intermediary, and virtually all but the Hartford group accepted it.

This system worked out well for many years, and I feel that the strength and the quality of the health care system in Connecticut is in part the result of the friendly and cooperative relationship between CBC and the health providers. Complications gradually emerged that made this partnership more difficult. Health care costs—particularly those of hospitals—rose, and Blue Cross became national, necessitating standard contracts which included medical services. This resulted in occasional friction with the separate Blue Shield plans. Available money, external regulations and controls, and competition assumed greater significance, so that relations between the voluntary hospital and what had been essentially a social program changed. Both hospitals and Blue Cross were now fighting for survival. I feel fortunate to have been associated with them when our working relationships were simply a genuine partnership of value and help to both parties.

GROUP PRACTICE

Although I knew that Blue Cross had been opposed by organized medicine in the 1930s and 1940s, the AMA's antipathy to group practice came as a surprise to me when I entered hospital administration. Stanford students and faculty watched the pioneering development of the Palo Alto Clinic by Tom Williams and its later expansion and formalization by Russell Lee. We accepted without question the Mayo, Lahey, Crile, and Joslin Clinics. I did not understand why the AMA later called the 1932 recommendation of the Committee on the Costs of Medical Care regarding group practice—particularly any prepaid financing mechanism— "socialized medicine." As a matter of fact, I find it difficult to understand what is meant when an individual or organization criticizes a medical or health program as "socialized medicine." The definitions of this term are usually fuzzy or self-serving. Too frequently it seems as if "socialized medicine" means any change from the existing system, especially if it is a program with which the doctor or organization disagrees.

In the late 1930s, Dr. MacLean was interested in developing an expanded clinic or group practice in Rochester. He asked me to explore the possibilities with our colleagues in Boston and New York. Our first introduction to the formal extension of a medical center's influence into a region came in 1940, when my wife and I visited the Pratt Diagnostic Clinic in Boston and met Samuel Proger and Abbie Dunks. I did not realize it at the time, but the Pratt Diagnostic Clinic's efforts to assure that the referring physician would always retain control over the care given his or her patient was also pioneering. The referral center was particularly careful to have the report and recommendations sent back to the private physician so as not to diminish his role.

The Boston meeting was followed by our first meeting with George Baehr of the Mt. Sinai Hospital Clinic in New York City. He introduced us to more examples of how traditional institutional and individual doctor-patient relationships might be extended beyond the hospital walls. At about the same time, we were visited in Rochester by Mildred Walker, who had been working with the Commonwealth Fund of New York City to sponsor small community hospitals in the Midwest and West. This was when Dr. Parnie Snoke and I developed the concept of regionalization associated with the teaching hospitals in Western New York. We spent much of our time over a two-year period becoming acquainted with the problems and needs of the hospitals in western New York State, and working closely with Lester Evans and Henry Southmayd of the Commonwealth Foundation in developing the philosophy of regionalization. To our delight, the foundation made its major grant to the Rochester area.

We quickly learned of the unpopularity of such radical ideas among our colleagues in organized medicine and on medical school faculties. The hospital regionalization program for western New York—which has provided the framework for successful collaborative effort for forty years—was not accepted by the faculty leaders of the University of Rochester Medical School until Albert Kaiser, a prominent pediatrician, became health officer in Rochester. He was able to bring to fruition our recommendations for a regionalization program, and he later told us that our work had provided additional background for the development of the Hill-Burton legislation (see chapter 8).

In the late 1930s and 1940s, a long, drawn-out battle took place between organized medicine and the Group Health Association in Washington, D.C. It was not settled until Assistant Attorney General Thurman Arnold charged the AMA and the local medical society with antitrust violations. His decision was upheld by the Supreme Court in 1943, which ruled that refusal of hospital privileges to physicians in group practice was illegal. This was a major turning point in organized medicine's opposition to this aspect of "socialized medicine." But skirmishes continued. The Health Insurance Plan of New York City (HIP) was started in March, 1947, in spite of many reservations about group practice. Years passed before many of the participating physicians would allow HIP members to come to their offices as if they were private patients—they were usually restricted to certain days or times. Even these tactics were regarded with suspicion by the doctors' colleagues in organized medicine. Many years later, Dr. Baehr described to me his indignation when he learned that the doctors in HIP were denied privileges in Staten Island hospitals on the insistence of the local medical society. He had to carry the fight to remove such restrictions to the New York State Legislature.

Those opposed to group practice sometimes went beyond simple professional pressure on doctors who did not conform to their beliefs. While my wife and I were attending a hospital meeting in San Francisco, a classmate invited many of our former colleagues from the medical school to a cocktail party. Among those present were Dr. and Mrs. Cecil Cutting. We were amazed to see them greeting classmates and friends—virtually neighbors of theirs in the San Francisco Bay area—as if they had not seen them for years. The reason was shockingly simple. Apparently Cecil had become associated with Sidney Garfield and Kaiser-Permanente. Organized medicine and many individual practicing physicians did not approve of the Permanente group practice, and as a result physicians and their spouses had engaged in what was essentially a planned program of social ostracism of those who were associated with Permanente.

Apparently I was an innocent living in a sheltered environment, for I continued to be surprised by the opposition of physician organizations to group practice and salary. Naively, I continued to dismiss these attitudes as aberrations, until I found myself embroiled in a similar confrontation in Connecticut. For this problem, involving Isidore Falk, group practice, and HMOs, I had only myself to blame.

Dr. Falk participated in the sessions I conducted for the AHA leading to the development of principles for hospital reimbursement. I came to respect his idealism and his broad social knowledge of medical care. When the faculty position in health care in the Yale University Department of Public Health opened up, I persuaded the dean of the School of Medicine and the chairman of the department to invite Dr. Falk to take the position. He came in 1961, and was soon responsible for major developments in the health care field in Connecticut.

I introduced Dr. Falk to Connecticut labor leaders, whom I respected—even though I consistently opposed them when they tried to organize the hospital. I was delighted when he and labor joined to start the first HMO in the state. But legislation was required to make the program possible and, as might be expected, a serious battle was engaged. It was led by the Connecticut State Medical Society, proving that organizational intransigence could encroach on my own turf. How much of the opposition was organized medicine's knee-jerk opposition to group practice and comprehensive, prepaid health insurance and how much was lingering resentment of Dr. Falk's pioneering work with the 1932 Committee on the Costs of Medical Care, I don't know. But reason prevailed, the legislation was passed, and the Long Wharf HMO has become one of the strongest in Connecticut.

Later in 1962, I was able to entice Richard Weinerman from the West Coast to head the ambulatory services division of the hospital and join the medical care faculty of the School of Public Health. From Drs. Falk and Weinerman I learned much about the potentials and pitfalls of group practice and HMOs. Dr. Weinerman was also a strong supporter of these programs. He had made a study of New Yorkers' preference for HIP and other groups or HMOs vs. Blue Cross and Blue Shield. To his surprise, a substantial majority preferred the more expensive Blue Cross and Blue

Shield. The reason was that patients valued their relationship with their own physician more than the lower cost of a group or HMO. Maintaining such a personal relationship has now become a basic principle of most group health insurance programs.

COMPONENTS OF THE HEALTH CARE SYSTEM

It is rather surprising how long it has taken many of us to recognize that health care involves organizing our programs to meet the ever-changing pattern of people's needs. The dominant voice when I was introduced to medicine was the doctor, and the dominant institution the hospital. I knew only patients who were so seriously ill that they had to be admitted to a hospital, and it took me years to recognize that there might be a number of other, interdependent components of a health care system, and that some sort of organized relationship between them was important to the efficiency and economy of the system, and important to the well-being of that patient in the hospital bed.

The Hospital

I became increasingly interested in combined approaches to health care through my introduction to health insurance and group practice. To most of us in health care, however, the important institution was still the acute care hospital, with its outpatient department and emergency room. Before I could begin to appreciate the importance of other components of the health system, I had to break out of my limited conception of the acute care hospital itself. I considered these institutions to be the most expensive, exciting, challenging, and therefore the most important part of the system. I accepted the traditional departmental organization of medical, surgical, pediatric, and obstetrical services and then only somewhat grudgingly added psychiatry. Next I learned of units for rehabilitation, long-term care, and intensive or specialized care of all varieties. Different visiting hours and meal customs, and patient councils in psychiatric and rehabilitation divisions had to be accepted. Parents were now living with their children in pediatrics, and rooming-in and natural childbirth programs, including birthing rooms, were flourishing. These increasingly specialized care units were the result of changes in professional approaches to different patient conditions, but also of a greater flexibility and understanding on the part of the administration.

As we developed these specialized care units, I learned more about the value of atmosphere and the individual needs of different kinds of patients. The rooming-in and natural childbirth innovations have already been mentioned. The change in the manner of caring for mothers after delivery came to my attention abruptly when the hospital received a flood of criticisms on patients' comment cards about the conditions in the bathrooms of the obstetric division. The Housekeeping Department and the director of nurses reported no change in personnel or daily census. I visited the division myself and agreed with the criticisms; wastebaskets in the bathrooms were overflowing and the rooms were cluttered. The head nurse thoughtfully remarked that the problem seemed to have coincided with the change in the rule on ambulation. The explanation became clearer—the custom in maternity had been bedrest and bedpans for seven days, then gradually increasing ambulation. The chief of obstetrics had changed this rule, and mothers were permitted to get up the first day after delivery. Suddenly, bathrooms, waste equipment, and housekeeping services intended for a twenty-eight-bed division with relatively few women walking about were completely inadequate for that same division with most of the women ambulatory. A simple change in medical treatment could affect the physical and personnel requirements of a hospital division.

Instituting the rehabilitation unit offered further education in the treatment of patients. Thomas Hines, the physiatrist responsible for this unit, insisted upon four-bed rooms—even for patients who had had relatively acute strokes. I wondered why (when I am sick, I want to be alone) until I visited the division. I watched patients with paralyses, amputations, and neurological and other incapacitating diseases taking an active role in explaining procedures and reassuring and encouraging new patients, and I saw clearly the tremendous contribution one patient could make to another with a similar problem. It is now widely recognized that many kinds of patients, from those who have had colostomies and mastectomies to those hospitalized for alchohol and drug abuse, benefit from communication with others who have similar conditions.

The care of children in the hospital also underwent revolutionary change during my career. When I was a resident in pediatrics at Stanford, visiting was allowed for two hours, twice a week. On the nights after visiting hours there was always a virtual epidemic of crying, restlessness, and even fever and other symptoms, leading us to discuss seriously abolishing visiting hours completely. In New Haven, under the influence of Drs. Powers, Senn, Gesell, and Solnit, I came to understand the value of relaxing the visiting rules in pediatrics. Soon parents were sleeping in children's rooms at night, some virtually living there and helping care for many of the children. And the children were happier and did better.

This philosophy has now extended to the delivery room. Although I was always supportive of rooming-in and natural childbirth, I was skeptical of allowing the father-to-be in the delivery room during birth. I knew that if I were a surgeon and an emergency occurred during an operation, I would not want an anxious or emotional relative present to distract me. Nor would I want to be interrupted by someone fainting at the sight of blood. Nevertheless, when the request was made to allow fathers to watch the delivery, I presented it to the medical board. It refused to grant permission. Some years later, I changed my mind and again made the proposal to the medical board. Again, the request was refused. I believe that I would have been far more persuasive if I had been able to describe to them the birth of the first child of my daughter-in-law and my second son. He was teaching in the Middle East Technical University in Ankara, Turkey. They decided on natural childbirth and both wanted him to be present at the birth. The university hospital refused, so they and their doctor found another Turkish hospital that would permit this. The look on the face of my daughter-in-law as she described the event and her feelings when her husband put her glasses on her and handed her their new little boy would have made me an enthusiastic supporter of the procedure if I had not been one already. Unfortunately, this event occurred some years later, or I would have led the charge against all doctors and hospital administrators who opposed this change in the rules.

Outpatient Services

The outpatient departments in large urban and teaching hospitals were all much the same. Most had large waiting rooms, usually with uncomfortable benches. Appointments were made for 8:00 A.M. or 1:00 P.M., after which the patient waited his or her turn. With rare exceptions, the medical staffing was also a standard pattern—the residents and students cared for the patients and the attending staff consulted. But hierarchy persisted here too. New physicians appointed to the faculty or the hospital's medical staff were expected to work at the clinics for several years before they were accepted as attending physicians on the inpatient service.

From my detached, medical point of view, the clinics at Stanford, Rochester, and New Haven seemed pretty good. Although I knew the pace was slow, I was satisfied that the patients' professional care was first class. In the late 1940s I was approached by two Yale graduate students, one in the Department of Sociology and the other in the School of Nursing, who proposed to write a joint thesis on the care of patients in our outpatient department and emergency room, from which they would write a paper for publication. They asked for my permission and for help in getting their paper accepted in a major hospital journal. I agreed. They did excellent, objective research and brought me their joint paper. Before sending it, as I had agreed, to a friend who was the editor of *Modern Hospital*, I read it and was appalled. There were no errors that I could discover; the thesis and article merely described our outpatient and emergency services as they were. It was an unflattering picture of how people were treated in the institution, whose two-tier approach to health care was made embarrassingly obvious.

After I read their work, I had to admit that their unflattering analysis was accurate. But I hated to see it described so baldly and publicly identified as the Out-Patient Department and Emergency Service of the Grace-New Haven Community Hospital. I decided that the only thing to do was to tell them honestly of my embarrassment and suggest that they delete the name and location of the institution and present it as a study of one of the university teaching centers on the East Coast. I thought that anyone who knew the various institutions would immediately identify it as Grace-New Haven—but at least the words would not be in print. The students agreed. A week later, on my way to Chicago, where I planned to deliver the manuscript to the journal editor, I shared a seat on the plane with Edwin Crosby, the director of the Johns Hopkins Hospital. I gave him the manuscript without any explanation. He read it and then turned to me in real indignation. Who were these authors? How did they get this information? Who in hell had given them permission to write about Johns Hopkins—and how had I gotten a copy of the manuscript? I reluctantly told him the truth. There was a small degree of comfort in this confirmation of what I already knew—that the shortcomings of my teaching hospital were not unique.

I was never satisfied with the separate clinic and private ambulatory facilities in the hospital, for they maintained the social separation between the clinic and private patients, even though the medical staff was the same. Consolidation admittedly would be difficult in such services as medicine, where a new patient was worked up by a student, a resident, and finally by the attending or consulting physician. However, in many specialty clinics the same examination, treatment, and follow-up procedures existed for both clinic and private patients. I started working on the various chiefs of service, and eventually managed to consolidate the clinic and private dermatology patients of Aaron Lerner and the tumor and x-ray therapy patients cared for by Morton Kligerman. I believed that the same staff, same physical facilities, and same amenities should be made available to all.

Emergency Services

Emergency services were always an exasperating problem to me. In my association with the hospitals at Stanford, Rochester, and New Haven, I was never much concerned about the quality of professional care that patients received. The problem was when and how people coming to the emergency division should be treated. The larger the institution with its proliferation of specialties, the greater were the possibilities for delay or confusion—but the greater was the chance of having a unique and potentially lifesaving service available.

One of the problems of the emergency division is the variety and intensity of patient conditions presenting themselves for treatment. Another is the problem of waiting for that treatment. Unless one has worked in such an environment, it is difficult to understand the delays. When a patient has a cut that is bleeding profusely and will require several stitches or has broken a wrist or an ankle, it seems to him or her to be an obvious emergency requiring immediate treatment. To the admitting staff, however, these situations are commonplace—a half dozen similar cases may appear in one evening. On the other hand, if an automobile accident produces seriously injured or dying patients with multiple injuries, virtually the entire emergency staff must concentrate upon lifesaving procedures. In these cases, a laceration or a broken bone must be a secondary episode, to be treated after the major problems are handled. There is also the problem of the perplexing case which requires consultation with one or more additional specialists who may not be immediately available. A twenty-minute wait may seem like hours to the patient or the family. Then there is the necessary red tape involved in obtaining name, address, previous hospital records, and the details of payment. Of all times to demand such information—when the patient is in pain, dripping blood, or just worried—the emergency situation is the worst. Yet, somehow, the information must be obtained.

Finally, there is the patient who has no identifiable malady but obviously needs temporary care. The solution to one such problem made history of a sort in Grace-New Haven. An elderly woman who lived alone had collapsed in her apartment and could not get up. Fortunately, she got the attention of neighbors and eventually ended up in the emergency room. Nothing could be found wrong with her. The residents felt she did not belong in the hospital, but there was no one else to take care of her.

I was awakened at midnight by a telephone call from a health officer, who indignantly demanded my intervention. I asked to talk to the resident. He agreed that she should not go home alone, and that no one could be found at that hour to care for her. But how could he admit her without a diagnosis? I asked if there was a bed available in the hospital until arrangements could be made the next morning. Yes—but how could he assign her to a service with no diagnosis? "That's simple," I said. "Admit her on the service "administration" and put me down as her attending physician." As far as I know, she remains the first and only patient ever admitted on the service of administration. It was a rather puzzling problem for our department of statistics. There is also little question that her discharge the next day was expedited.

Despite its important work and good intentions, the emergency department seemed always to attract complaints about waiting, overcharging, unnecessary procedures, paperwork, and incorrect diagnoses. I tried all types of approaches to improve the reputation of our emergency services. First was to employ a topflight surgeon to run the ER. He expedited patient care, but he wasn't happy administering and expediting rather than doing surgery, his first love. And he could not work out a pattern by which he was not considered a favored competitor by his surgical colleagues.

I then asked a distinguished retired physician to take charge. This was quite successful, as was the employment of a compassionate senior administrative nurse. Both were able to emphasize to the staff the value of explaining the emergency service situation to the patients. Most patients do not mind the wait if they understand its reason and know that they are not forgotten. We also started a triage system, by which the seriously ill were routed to immediate care and the others to another part of the facility. The care of the acutely ill was easily dealt with, but remembering to explain and expedite the care of the nonemergency patient was a constant problem. The present custom, with hospitals employing groups of physicians solely for emergency care, may be a better solution, although it is expensive. I do not know whether this type of care is professionally satisfying as a career, but many physicians are choosing this now-recognized specialty.

I was first introduced to the specialized role of the hospital emergency service as part of an organized acute trauma program when I was the coordinator of health services in Illinois. Bruce Flashner and David Boyd had come to me in 1970 with an idea to expand and certify regional trauma services. Dr. Flashner, who was an assistant of mine in the State Office, had been head of the Trauma and Emergency Service at Cook County Hospital, with which Dr. Boyd was still involved. My wife and I had been profoundly impressed with that emergency service, particularly as we heard so many knowledgeable persons declare that, if they were seriously injured, this was the institution and the service to which they wanted to be taken. Drs. Boyd and Flashner wanted to set up a regional system of regional trauma centers in Illinois. Special training and facilities would be required, and the state would arrange communication and transportation (by ambulance or helicopter) so that patients could be quickly transferred and treated. Their ideas fascinated me and I agreed to present the program to the governor and other appropriate people. Drs. Flashner and Boyd, with the help of my wife, Dr. Parnie, prepared a formal proposal. Within a short time, the Illinois Trauma Center Program was launched, and from that came the National Trauma Center Program, of which David Boyd became the administrative chief in HEW and later HHS (Health and Human Services).

Short-Term Service Centers

In planning the medical center in New Haven in the early 1960s, we explored the possibility of setting up separate service centers for minor procedures or emergencies. It seemed safer and more convenient for these facilities to be closely associated with the medical center. We hoped to program and staff them in such a way that minor cases could be seen promptly while major cases were shifted into the mainstream of highly sophisticated care. We also planned a short-term elective procedure unit in which patients could be treated, observed, and then sent home the same day with adequate follow-up. Associated with this unit, in an adjacent office building, were to be facilities for community physicians. They would thus be able not only to care easily for their hospital patients, but also to have these minor procedure centers available. In addition to these proposed new service centers, which now are called "surgicenters" or "emergicenters," we also hoped to incorporate other services and facilities that a number of other medical centers throughout the country were developing. These included doctors' offices, parking, motels and restaurants for families and visitors and out-of-town patients, and a bank and a pharmacy.

The planned medical center did not emerge in the early 1960s for a number of reasons, some problems of politics and timing, some involving town-and-gown conflicts. Another problem that now must be faced in this type of operation is accurate separation of the costs of the acute-care and the minor services. It is tempting to shift overhead costs back and forth, depending on the type of reimbursement and cost analyses.

Some years later, a medical office and procedure building was constructed downtown with many of the short-stay, minor procedure facilities incorporated into the services offered. It is well run and, fortunately, large enough to handle most of the emergencies that may arise. However, the physician responsible for the facility frankly admitted that it probably would not have been built if our original plans had come to fruition. Now, almost twenty-five years later, both the medical center and the downtown medical office building are proposing motel facilities. I was obviously a poor salesman.

The medical center did expand in the late 1960s to sponsor "satellite" neighborhood health centers in nearby communities. Our objective was to provide facilities to take the place of the hospital outpatient department and in which community residents would have a voice. The medical center was to provide the necessary professional services. We were slower to implement this than institutions like Tufts and Johns Hopkins. But by the end of the 1960s the Hill Health Center was established, with the assistance of the Connecticut Regional Medical Program and the Yale Medical School, and has continued to serve the area.

STATEWIDE HEALTH PLANNING

The shift of my attention beyond the hospital walls came slowly. I was faced daily with administrative crises in making two hospitals in New Haven function as one. Moreover, during the 1940s and 1950s, the acute-care general hospitals, with its developing subdivisions and its outpatient and emergency departments, seemed already to be a major influence on the health care system. Connecticut's hospitals were independent, voluntary, community institutions, none with fewer than fifty beds, and Connecticut was the only state whose hospitals were all accredited by the JCAH. There was little overt competition, even between hospitals in the same city. The state was not demonstrably overbedded, costs appeared to be within reason, and the relationships among the hospitals, Blue Cross, commercial insurance companies, and the state health and social agencies were friendly and cooperative.

My first step toward extending the influence of the hospital and medical center was still institutional. I was formally asked by Governor Lodge in April, 1952, to work with his administrative assistant, Colonel Raymond Watt, to develop recommendations for a more integrated state mental health department, in which the commissioner would have more clearcut authority. I was also asked to plan a decentralization of state mental health care with the programs to be associated with acute-care general hospitals. I received most of my ideas from Theodore Lidz and Fritz Redlich of the Department of Psychiatry of the Yale Medical School, and from Wilfred Bloomberg, the commissioner of Mental Health, whose responsibilites were limited and ill-defined.

In due course I submitted a carefully written series of recommendations to Colonel Watt. The action taken not only formalized the position and responsibility of the commissioner of mental health in Connecticut, but also established the process which created the first state mental health adjunct institution. It was built next to the Yale-New Haven Hospital and was in close professional relationship with the Department of Psychiatry. It provided a valuable extension of state mental health resources in the local area and was emulated in Hartford, whose institution was associated with the University of Connecticut Medical Center, and in Bridgeport. A program to regionalize other mental health facilities statewide was also developed.

My next involvement with statewide health planning involved an attempt to improve planning for hospitals. This grew out of my previous experience developing a mental health program, the cooperative attitude of the CHA member hospitals and state agencies, and my growing understanding of the national health scene through my involvement with the AHA. During the late 1950s, it became apparent that local, regional, and statewide health planning was inadequate. I was dissatisfied with the rather unimaginative process by which the state distributed its federal Hill-Burton funds each year. I had no personal reason for this belief, for I always had a legitimate project to present, and it was always approved for a grant. But there was little evident effort to use those funds or Connecticut's considerable leadership potential in health for statewide planning.

In 1960 I approached Governor Abraham Ribicoff about a health planning commission for the state. He approved of the idea and appointed a planning committee for this before accepting the secretaryship of HEW. As the committee explored the state's health problems and programs, I was struck by the fragmentation of the private resources and organizations concerned with health and social welfare in the state, and the corresponding fragmentation of the state and federal agencies with which we in the health field were dealing. (I fear this phenomenon still exists.) After about two years of discussion, the committee formally recommended to the governor that the state sponsor an independent, broadly representative hospital planning agency that could make recommendations to the Department of Health's Hill-Burton Agency and to the hospitals—although the agency itself could not have the power of formal approval. The recommendations were torpedoed at the last minute because the State Medical Society and the commissioner of health recommended disapproval to Governor Ribicoff's successor, John Dempsey. I was rather stunned when the commissioner of health recommended disapproval, inasmuch as he had been a member of the planning committee for two years, and we had spent many months rewriting the report to meet his objections. However, I was also sympathetic to the governor's position on an issue that he had inherited and which was now opposed by his own commissioner. So I suggested that I draft a letter for the Governor to send to me. At his request, I drafted one describing the complexities of such an organization and recommending that it be done on a voluntary basis, rather than under the auspices of the state. Governor Dempsey returned the letter to me officially a few days later, and in 1965 the Connecticut Hospital Planning Commission was formed. It was delayed because of the reservations of a number of Connecticut hospitals about accepting federal funds for a program that they believed should be their own business. They finally agreed to guarantee financial support for at least two years, with no strings attached, and so long as only a minority of the board were administrators of hospitals. The commissioner of health and members of the medical society became members of the planning commission, and within a short time the Hill-Burton Agency was asking the voluntary planning body for its recommendations on Hill-Burton requests. Connecticut Blue Cross also began to require the commission's approval before it would accept new construction depreciation expenses for reimbursement. The commission thus became a nongovernmental Certificate of Need agency!

CONTINUUM OF CARE AND REGIONAL PLANNING

We had been slow in extending our services beyond the medical center until the mid-1960s—the only exception was the rather laborious development of the Hill Health Center. This experience, as well as the programs being initiated in many other medical centers throughout the country, brought home to me how insular our thinking and planning in these medical centers could become. I began to think more seriously of the responsibility of the hospital and the medical center for health activities outside our immediate environment. One important consideration was that many health-care needs could be met more easily and cheaply outside the hospital.

I gradually came to think that our planning should be based upon the continuum of health care philosophy, which sees a person as existing in an ever-changing state of health, for which all types of services or facilities should be available. Our challenge was to organize the system so that people could obtain the necessary services easily, promptly, and as inexpensively as possible. When I presented my ideas to my hospital colleagues in 1961, I showed graphically the interrelationship of the short-term hospital, the long-term hospital, the nursing home, ambulatory care resources, and home care. I indicated how the patient could shift from one type of care to another, depending upon his or her condition.

During this period little effort was being made to combine institutions or even services on a regional or statewide basis. The primary exception was group purchasing, in which hospitals in a relatively large area in the East used the services of the Hospital Bureau of New York City. Over the years, the CHA expanded the services it provided to its member institutions, but this was still on the initiative of the individual institution—regional planning was not involved. Following the example of some other regions, I invited a consultant to advise on the possibility of an independent regional laundry for Yale-New Haven and a number of neighboring hospitals. The projections indicated that the savings per pound to our institution would be small, because of our large volume, but the smaller institutions would realize substantially greater savings. There were additional savings on replacement of equipment in several hospitals, as well as the elimination of the need for a laundry in a new hospital that was being built. Yale-New Haven also profited from the release of a large amount of valuable space. But all our thinking was still restricted to how independent institutions might share services.

By the mid-1960s, I had had the opportunity to consult with a number of Connecticut hospitals on various building projects. I was struck with the fact that virtually every hospital and community expected to have every professional service, whether or not the demand warranted it, whether or not the service could be operated economically and with high standards. This included pediatrics, obstetrics, high voltage x-ray therapy, complex laboratory procedures, and many of the more esoteric surgical specialties. In several regions, two hospitals less than ten miles apart operated obstetrical hospitals at 40–50 percent occupancy. I started pointing out the possibility of combining such services in one hospital or the other. I even had an associate calculate the average number of empty obstetrical beds in Yale-New Haven and St. Raphael. Sister Louise and I determined that each of our institutions could free about thirty beds for some other specialty if we were to combine our obstetrical medical staffs, continue to maintain the two obstetrical service units, but use the beds of both facilities interchangeably. All but four doctors already had privileges in both hospitals, and, of these four, two were retiring and the other two were acceptable to both institutions. We recognized the potential problems of a combined Catholic and non-Catholic obstetrical service, but felt that with an attitude of flexibility in the two hospital units, the beliefs of the patients, doctors, and institutions could be respected. I regret that I left Yale-New Haven before Sister Louise and I had a chance to explore seriously this radical idea with our medical staffs, boards, and patients. It is hard to imagine it really happening.

I continued to be attracted by the possibility of combining services and facilities to save personnel, space, and money through a management and planning organization for the thirty-five voluntary hospitals in Connecticut. By the mid-1960s, operational costs for the Connecticut voluntary hospitals were approximately $500 million a year. They are now approaching $1.75 billion a year. A number of my colleagues and I spent many hours investigating the savings that might result if there were just one voluntary hospital system in Connecticut to coordinate the current hospitals needed—probably fewer than the current thirty-five. Such a system would unify standards of materials, purchasing, and management, and clinical services would be available on the basis of patient need, not tradition. In this mid-1960s pipe dream, we blithely calculated that the annual savings would amount to 10 percent, or fifty million dollars. One can only conjecture on the possible savings today.

It is a tribute to the CHA leadership that the organization has been gingerly but intelligently exploring the idea of a Connecticut hospital system over the past two years. This could restructure and strengthen the state's voluntary hospital system. Unfortunately, the national corporate multihospital system has appeared so attractive that a number of hospitals in the state have joined the Voluntary Hospitals of America, which in turn prompted other Connecticut institutions to become affiliated with another hospital group. The CHA is now exploring means of coordinating what may well be battling giants with the remaining community hospitals. This may be music to the ears of competition advocates, but will it be the best for our overall health care system?

Since 1965, I have viewed with great interest the practical realization of my dreams as hospital corporations have emerged. I first became aware of this as I watched the growth of the Samaritan Health System in Arizona. I always enjoyed teasing Steve Morris, its CEO, because, although their title emphasized the term "Health System," it was really a corporation of hospitals only.

I confess that I was somewhat startled when they went to another corporate level, which included not only voluntary, nonprofit hospital organizations, but also profit-making enterprises. Five of these systems (Samaritan, Lutheran, Inter-Mountain, Southwest Community, and Adventists), along with seven other similar systems, then created a nonprofit entity which was formally institutionalized in 1982 as the Associated Hospital Systems, with Monte DuVal as its first President. In 1984, they changed their name to the Associated Health Systems! On a somewhat parallel track, another group of hospitals and systems formed the United Health Care Systems in Kansas City, and, as what appeared to be the inevitable next step, joined with the Associated Health Systems to form the American Health Care Systems. This now numbers 34 systems. They own, lease, or manage 495 hospitals and render direct services by contract to another 950 affiliates. They cover 44 states and their revenue is approximately $14 billion annually. When one considers the growth of other institutional giants, such as the Voluntary Hospitals of America, and the tremendous proprietary chains, such as the Hospital Corporation of America and Humana, there is little question that providing health care has become big business. The American Health Care Systems has also developed an interesting, nonprofit division, now located in Washington, with Dr. DuVal as its president and CEO. It is concerned with educational activities, research into the operation and characteristics of multihospital systems, and development and advocacy of policy positions favorable to development of multi-hospital systems. This may be very helpful both to the hospitals and to the government. However, as the number of hospital lobbying groups grows (there are now more than fifteen separate organizations in Washington), fragmentation threatens to dilute the effectiveness of the organization I consider most important, the AHA. Opposing interests will happily use the opportunity to "divide and conquer."

Problems of efficiency of operation, central purchasing, attracting the best talent in the increasingly competitive health business, generating additional revenue through profit enterprises, and the need for large amounts of capital at good interest rates have led to these developments. And the political influence that large health corporations can wield has not been overlooked. These are some of the reasons for the phenomenal growth of the for-profit hospitals, nursing homes, organizations of "surgicenters" and "emergicenters," as well as for the combining of nonprofit and for-profit enterprises. The dangers of hospitals as big business are suggested in the title of an article by Arnold Relman, editor of the *New England Journal of Medicine*: "The Medical-Industrial Complex."[2] Dr. Relman's medical-industrial complex is not limited to the profit-making health or hospital corporations. As I have noted, nonprofit, voluntary supercorporations also cannot avoid the problems that come with increas-

2. A. S. Relman, "The New Medical-Industrial Complex," *New England Journal of Medicine* 303 (1980), 963–70.

ing size, levels of authority and responsibility, and operations that mount to the billions of dollars. I also fear that, like other big business, the hospital systems will be in constant flux based not on the interests of the individual patient or the community, but on the influence of the dollar.

I do not envy either my colleagues in health care and administration or the patients (who are the public) as they face the future. Concern about the increasing health costs is growing, and, of course, it is the public that must pay. Political activity will increase. Proposals including state rate commissions, controlling the health industry as if it were a utility or a government responsibility, will be considered at the state and federal levels. The Arizona effort to control hospitals through the utility model failed in 1984, but the issue will undoubtedly recur. In the spring of 1984, Connecticut found the State Cost Commission, the commercial insurance companies, and private industry pitted against the hospitals, the physicians, and Blue Cross, on the method of hospital reimbursement. This eventually resulted in compromise legislation. But I deplore confrontation as a method of solving problems. I have always tried to get all parties together to work out the best solutions for the patient—which is not just the solution in the middle. For complex problems, the success rate of the confrontational method—political maneuvering, debate, legislation, and regulation—is abysmally poor.

The primary responsibility of the health care system is the health and welfare of the individual patient in the context of his or her family, environment, and community. We must not lose sight of this primary responsibility as we enter the exciting world of organization, corporations, for-profit and nonprofit subsidiaries, and capital expansion and construction. If giant health corporations become like other giant corporations, preoccupied with the balance sheet, competition, shareholder dividends, and exciting new ventures, the patient will be lost in the shuffle. This is particularly true if primary attention is given to the horizontal development of the expensive, impressive institutional edifice rather than vertical organizations concerned with a continuum of care. As I discovered twenty years ago, voluntary community resources such as hospitals, home health, and visiting nurse agencies are a source of local community pride and protectiveness, part of an American town tradition. Because of this, all of my planning has involved preserving local participation and responsibility. I believe that fundamental to any form of consolidation is to take the greatest advantage of local advisory boards and citizen participation, as well as to stimulate coordination and cooperation.

I cannot, of course, disagree with organizational changes that will eliminate duplication and waste, promote efficiency, and provide more services for people at less cost. I can only point out to the corporate planners and managers that the programs we are operating, and the objectives we piously support, must yield the best care possible for people. We must not only think of the patient as a person but must also create mechanisms and organization that clearly define authority and responsibility for the primary goal of the best care for each patient. How do you combine multi-billion-dollar, many-tiered supercorporations, the balance sheet, and the philosophy of competition with a mechanism that will ensure that someone has identifiable responsibility for that individual patient being cared for in that single institution at the lowest rung of the corporate ladder?

HEALTH SERVICES PLUS SOCIAL SERVICES
EQUALS HUMAN SERVICES

Beyond the big business challenge is another social phenomenon that will really complicate our corporate planners and organizational enrepreneurs as they start planning, reorganizing, and expanding the brave new world of multi-corporations for health services. This is the fact that health services and social services for people are intimately related. I did not recognize this phenomenon during my years in hospital administration in Rochester or New Haven. Not until I embarked upon my next postgraduate educational period, from 1969 to 1973, as coordinator for health services for Illinois, did I learn that society (and I) should be concerned about people—but not just as patients.

When I arrived in Illinois, I considered myself a health professional, and, naturally, wanted to be of the greatest assistance to the governor in his health responsibilities. I became acquainted with the directors and division heads of Public Health, Mental Health, Public Welfare, Children and Family Services, Aging, Crippled Children's Services, and so on, and quickly became aware of the diversity of state departments that were concerned with one or another aspect of health. I hoped to simplify the state administrative organization, and for almost twelve months I patiently explored with each director and his or her senior department heads those interests or activities in the department that were related to health. My ultimate objective was to create a single health department that would bring together all the apparently fragmented divisions.

The directors and department heads were cooperative and honest. I respected them as professionals in their own fields, and they knew that I did not want to take over their departments or take away their jobs. But the director of Mental Health, Albert Glass, frankly pointed out the difficulty of separating health from other activities. "How can I do it?" he asked. "I have mental patients in institutions, in halfway homes, or discharged under supervision. I am concerned with their social situation, their jobs, their housing, and their orientation to society. I cannot separate health from these other factors." The director of Children and Family Services was equally explicit. "Of course I am concerned about children's health, but I am also concerned about their housing, education, nutrition, and family environment. I cannot separate health from all these other factors." The same problem obviously beset the divisions concerned with aging, and the welfare director too reminded me that health was only one aspect of the overall welfare of his charges. Within my first year in Illinois, I made a 180-degree turn, replacing my emphasis on health with one on health and social services. I found that I, too, could not separate health from housing, environment, nutrition, education, and income. This is a philosophy that I brought back from Illinois. It is the primary reason I disagree with colleagues who advocate further division of the original HEW (now HHS). As I will discuss in more detail in chapter 9, I support a major cabinet division in the state government for health and human services.

Finally, the prevention of disease and the restriction of other avoidable causes of death or illness—guns, drunken driving, tobacco, industrial hazards, and drugs—should not be left to zealots or special interests. They are the responsibility of society and its representatives—if we can protect *them* from these same zealots! But deaths from these causes are sometimes scarcely noticed in comparison to untoward deaths in hospitals. Health and social customs are interrelated and our approach to the problems of corporate organization, salaries, regulation, and costs must take into account this interweaving.

8

Reimbursement and Cost Containment, Planning, Regulation, and Control

The issue of controls for the delivery and financing of health care was a minor one early in the century. Isolated voices and organizations raised questions about quality and access and suggested an increased government role, but little was done. Organized medicine fiercely opposed any change in the status quo of individual patient-physician relationships and fee-for-service professional practice. Any suggested change, whatever it might be, was referred to as "socialized medicine," whose evils were axiomatically abhorred. The effect of change upon the physician's pocketbook was tacitly ignored.

As the health care delivery system became more complex, health costs, reimbursement formulae, available money, and control of expenditure assumed greater importance. Planning, priorities, health care as a right or as a privilege, nonprofit and profit enterprise vs. government-controlled medicine, and competition all became important components in the attempts to develop a national health policy—which has still not been clearly defined. When the actual costs for health care and the percentage of the GNP spent on health care grew to what many consider to be astronomical proportions, voices again called for specific regulation and control of the industry. Both locally and nationally, they could not avoid emphasizing money. One has only to look at the figures—over $350 billion spent on health nationally in 1984, the 1986 budget of $332.9 billion and the 1987 budget of $345.6 billion for the Department of Health and
128

Human Services (which represents only a part of government spending for health)—to understand this interest. During my ten years in Rochester (1937–1946), hospital costs and payment for hospital care were not considered great problems. Several factors—the prevailing philosophy of philanthropy, the overcharging of private patients to subsidize ward patients, the shameless exploitation of the student nurse and other hospital personnel, who received low or no pay, and the beginnings of the technological explosion in health care—helped keep hospital costs from becoming a big problem. If patients could pay the full rate or had insurance, they were private; if they could pay less, they were, as it was termed in Rochester, "service." Others entered the RMH section of SMH or went to the Monroe County Hospital. Hospital rates were as low as possible; the deficit was made up by the university endowment.

When I came to New Haven in 1946, I faced the economic facts of life in a combination teaching, community, and municipal hospital with a negligible endowment. For over a century, this institution had cared for all who came to its doors. I was impressed with this tradition—it was one of the primary reasons I accepted the position there. However, costs were rising. We were slowly stopping the exploitation of student nurses and other personnel. And I was working with the board and Yale University to end our dependence on the annual subsidy from the university. We had no recourse but to get adequate reimbursement for the care that we provided, unless we wanted to watch the institution go broke.

At this time, the state and town welfare departments paid four dollars a day for care that cost the hospital approximately ten dollars. About 25 percent of the patients were on welfare. Another 20 percent were "working poor," self-supporting but with no way to pay for major health care—particularly when the family wage earner was sick. The heads of the welfare services in most of the 169 towns and cities in Connecticut had widely varying ideas on morality, illness, and their welfare responsibility. For example, the admitting officers often told me that one town or another would refuse to pay for the care of an unmarried pregnant woman—particularly if she were foreign or black. We took care of these patients, but financial responsibility for them was only slowly and reluctantly accepted by the welfare officers—primarily because of several landmark court decisions in Connecticut, some of which were initiated by Grace-New Haven before and after I came.

Some of the changes in attitude were, I am sure, the result of the gradual shifting of financial responsibility from towns to the state. I welcomed this, not only because the state was able to attract several competent, socially oriented professionals to its welfare and social service departments, but also because many small towns in Connecticut would have had their welfare budget completely wiped out by one long hospital stay. But the locus of welfare responsibility was not my gravest financial concern. Rather, it was reconciling the daily payment for welfare patients with the cost. This was especially important for Grace-New Haven, which had the highest percentage of welfare patients in the state. I saw no alternative but to press for realistic reimbursement, and I started a state-wide effort. Eventually, cost-basis reimbursement went national. Hailed as revolutionary at the time, it is now assailed by government and medical economists, and even by some doctors (even surgeons, who are not notorious for their frugality). These critics argue that cost-based reimbursement has given hospitals and medical centers free rein to increase costs without attempting to curtail them by means of efficient operation. I suspect that, had any of these critics been on the staff of Grace-New Haven during the late 1940s, he or she would have been just as concerned as I was about the continued existence of the hospital.

My first effort to obtain adequate payment was made through a committee that I persuaded the governor to appoint in 1948. Senator Robert E. Parsons was the chairman, and he was assisted by the commissioner of welfare, his welfare medical director, and Lewis Johnson, the acting controller of the New Britain Memorial Hospital. (Mr. Johnson believes he was appointed because his hospital was the only one in Connecticut that made money under the low state welfare payments.) I represented the state's hospitals. The committee recommended legislation to provide cost-based payment for welfare patients, using the AHA chart of accounts as the basis for calculation of costs. This was what I advocated, and I have often wondered whether the decision was due to my persuasiveness or to the suggestion of Mr. Johnson, the state's supposedly unbiased expert, who urged that the state pay the hospital's published rates—which are routinely much higher than costs. That, not surprisingly, seemed entirely too much to the rest of the committee and the legislature, and so we compromised on cost or charges, whichever was lower. This principle has existed for many years. The committee also recommended the creation of a Hospital Cost Commission, made up of the commissioners of health, mental health, welfare, and finance, and a small review staff. Costs were first to be audited by the hospitals' own auditors, then by the Connecticut Hospital Association, and finally by the Connecticut State Hospital Cost Commission.

This was a major step forward in state welfare reimbursement, and, although Connecticut was the point state, my friends and associates in Massachusetts, New York, and Maryland proved of great help. In constant communication, we traded ideas, techniques, modifications, and procedures. Connecticut passed the law in 1949, with a flat per-diem payment of ten dollars a day for the first two years, giving the new cost commission and the hospitals time to gear up for the program. In 1951, state per-diem payments to the hospitals for inpatient care were based on actual cost.

Although the underlying principle had already been accepted by the Emergency Maternal and Infant Care program (EMIC), the Veterans' Administration (VA), and the servicemen's dependents' health care program (now CHAMPUS), no formal statement outlining which cost factor should be included had ever been introduced or accepted for a nation-wide program. As chairman of the AHA Council on Prepayment and Reimbursement, I held a meeting in 1951 to develop principles for a national reimbursement program. Innocently, I invited representatives of every interest group I could think of. Besides hospitals and Blue Cross, we included representatives from the United Auto Workers and the United Mine Workers, the Health Insurance Plan of New York City, the VA, the U.S. Children's Bureau, the Catholic and Protestant hospital associations, and commercial insurance. I recall none from industry, but at that time industry was not particularly interested.

About one-half hour after the two-day session started, it seemed to be turning into a disaster. I knew only a little about parliamentary rules of running a meeting, but I soon found myself among parliamentary pros like Isidore Falk, and just about every conceivable special pleader and nitpicker. There were immediately motions and amendments. Then we moved on to amendments to amendments, points of order, debates over procedures, and challenges of numbers, rules, intents, and meaning. I became as confused as everyone else about what was happening, and I could see the session ending in a shambles.

When it became obvious that the special pleaders would keep us from doing anything, I interrupted the session. I described the situation as I saw it and the difficulty of accomplishing anything constructive in this manner. I then told the group that we would proceed according to Snoke's rules of order. I would introduce the subject and encourage free and open discussion. When I decided that I had heard enough of the issue, I would stop the discussion, write up a motion and offer it, listen to the discussion, either change the motion or leave it, and put it to a vote. Anyone who did not like this procedure could go home—or I would. They were all so tired of the procedural morass that, to my surprise and pleasure, they all accepted. At the end of two days, we had an acceptable first draft. The AHA distributed it widely to various agencies over the next year, and in

January, 1953, we met for a second time. From this, the principles of hospital cost reimbursement went to the AHA board of trustees and House of Delegates and were formally adopted in September, 1953. For years, most third-party agencies accepted them as a basis for hospital cost reimbursement. At the dinner at the end of the second session, after we had all congratulated ourselves on our accomplishment, Donald McGowan, the primary spokesman for the Catholic hospitals and a respected member of the AHA board of trustees, arose and made a flowery speech praising the session's accomplishments and my officiating. He then gave me an elaborately wrapped present. Both my wife and I knew exactly what it was—a copy of "Robert's Rules of Order."

After the development of the principle of cost-based payment, I had a series of long conversations with Basil MacLean. We both believed this type of reimbursement was proper and necessary at the time for both hospital and third parties. But we knew it would be abused and believed that controls would be necessary. As long as this reimbursement covered only a minority of the patient load, the hospital would have incentives for economy and efficiency, because its direct billings could not be out of line with other hospitals. But, as the percentage of patients for whom the hospitals received payment on a cost basis grew, the incentive for efficiency and cost control would lose strength. Basil MacLean and I searched for some type of control that would not grant us a blank check. It is perhaps worth noting that my former student, associate, and academic colleague, John Thompson, along with Robert Fetter, played a major role in the development of DRGS, the newest approach to reimbursement as a means of cost containment. The Diagnostic Related Groups have been widely accepted, have helped bring into focus the cost factors of procedures and tests, as well as the patient's length of stay in the acute care hospital, the most expensive unit of the health care system.

I tried in the 1960s to promote ambulatory care service units. I did not succeed in New Haven, but many other medical centers did. I talked for years about the "continuum of care" in various levels of facilities. But only when I later learned more about the potentials of less expensive care at home or in a nursing home did I fully see the practical possibilities of a better and cheaper health care system. This type of thinking is stimulated by DRGS, although I doubt whether the developers of DRGS had the broader aspects of the continuum of care in mind. Rather, they considered the expense of hospital care. The DRG principles require the physician and the institution to consider carefully the cost of caring for a specific patient in relation to his or her disease, the procedures or tests ordered, the type of facility required, and the duration of stay. The result has been a demonstrable decrease in patients' length of stay in many hospitals.

But I worry chiefly about the future. Our federal programs are not noted for their simplicity, consistency, equity, or longevity. Our problems are only beginning and respected administrators and economists are challenging the principles. Stuart Altman, for example, describes a phenomenon called "DRG Creep."[1] He points out that, in attempting to calculate hospitals' DRG reimbursement limits as fairly as possible, Congress has adopted a complicated system of case-mix adjustments. Some believe these complications make the DRG system susceptible to manipulation, or, as Altman puts it, easily "gamed." "Small games can be tolerated, but if the gaming rate should approach the 10% to 15% level, the system will not achieve its goal." Alain C. Enthoven and Roger G. Noll are even less sanguine about the long-term success of DRGS.[2] Part of their criticism is directed toward the premise upon which the DRG approach is based. They also propose another system, based upon competition, and argue that this has a better chance to solve all problems and silence all doubters.

The complexities of organization, administration, and financing health care will challenge our best minds for years to come. The academic experts at Yale nonchalantly solve each challenge by some seemingly simple adjustment that only they understand. I applaud the effort, but I am still uncomfortable for the future. However, in the meantime, the pressure to decrease the number of acute care hospital beds—and even hospitals—as well as involving the doctor in the economic risks of health care are major contributions for which we have the DRG principles to thank.

Physicians' share of fiscal responsibility is unfortunately not clearly emphasized in the 1986 article by McMahon, Fetter, Freeman, and Thompson, "Hospital Matrix Management."[3] We must be frequently reminded of the physician's contribution to the cost of the patient's hospital stay. To my disappointment, their article seemed to assign the hospital and its administrator the narrow role of assuring efficiency and economy of the "intermediate products" of the institutional operation, along with "efficiency of production." The overall care of the patient, the responsibility of the hospital board and the CEO for this care, and the ways physicians share in the fiscal and professional results of the hospital's operation were not addressed in this new matrix organization.

I have a final word of caution regarding the use of DRGS. While they stimulate more prudent use of the most expensive component of the

1. S. H. Altman, "The American Health Care System: A Rube Goldberg Apparatus," The Esselstyn "Spirit of Man" Lecture, June 12, 1984.

2. A. C. Enthoven and R. G. Noll, "Prospective Payment: Will It Solve Medicare's Financial Problems?" *Issues in Science and Technology* (Fall 1984), 106–16.

3. L. F. McMahon et al., "Hospital Matrix Management and DRG-Based Prospective Payment," *Hospital and Health Services Administration* (January-February 1986), 62–85.

health care system, the acute care hospital, they are fundamentally epi-
sodic in approach. Yet the patient goes through various conditions of
illness and health and requires consideration in terms of a continuum of
care. The little man in the statue "Discharged Cured" may have received
the exact type of treatment and length of stay in the acute-care hospital
that the DRG standards define, but society's responsibility for him does not
end when the DRG formula has been met. The DRG payment system may
be utilized very efficiently and economically to discharge the elderly
patient, but what happens next? Skilled nursing home care, immediate
care facilities, long-term nursing homes, and home health care as well as
hospices are all components of the continuum of care for that elderly
person. I know that John Thompson and Robert Fetter are aware of the
continuing needs of many patients. Their DRG approach for hospitals
should not be used as an excuse to ignore these needs. We also must
recognize that the developing system of financing health care providers—
primarily stimulated by the DRG approach—does not automatically result
in a sound and equitable health system. Some hospitals and health
agencies are doing embarrassingly well financially, while other important
and necessary health resources are fighting for survival. Our health and
welfare problems and the needs of people cannot be solved by a reimbursement policy alone.

HOSPITAL CHARGES

Hospital charges for individual services were, of course, the time-honored means by which the hospitals received reimbursement. Hospitals
obviously needed income to pay for their expenses and, when necessary,
to underwrite the care of the poor. The specific amount charged for
individual items in the hospital bill has never been easy to explain or
defend. Room charges usually included the standard "hotel" maintenance items, administration, food, and overhead, as well as the professional charge for nursing. These charges were almost always substantially
below cost, and charges for special services were usually above cost.
Special services included drugs, operating rooms, special procedures,
and the hospital-based professional services such as radiology, anesthesiology, and pathology. Administrators hoped the charges for the special
services would make up for the loss incurred by room and nursing, plus
the additional losses from bad debts and free care.

    Because of my continuing difficulties with the problem of salary for
hospital-based professionals, I was particularly watchful over the charges
for these services. I did not want to lend any support to the charge that the

hospital profited from salaried radiologists, pathologists, or anesthesiologists. It was not easy to answer these criticisms because, traditionally, charges for such hospital-based services had been substantially above costs.

In anesthesiology, we kept the hospital charges stable as salaries and other costs increased. When the annual audit showed a loss in the Department of Anesthesia, I was delighted and told everyone who would listen. Clinical pathology was not too much of a problem—we tried to pay the professional staff fairly and charged less than the commercial laboratories. I never solved the radiology problem. Our salary scales for radiologists were the same as or higher than those for the full-time medical school faculty, but the hospital still turned a profit in the department. I tried to lower charges, but both our full-time radiologists and many of the community practitioners complained that this would create an embarrassing disparity between our hospital's charges and the rates charged in the community and in the other hospital. In this case I let my respect for the radiologists take precedence over the principle of keeping costs down. Also, as the hospital was paid on a cost basis by most third parties, the charges applied only to ambulatory service patients and those covered by commercial insurance. Today, I regret that the savings to the patient for the services of most hospital-based specialties are negligible. In many teaching hospitals the medical school now administers the specialty services, and charges are very close to those of private practitioners. A final comment on charges: the traditional multiple page bill listing individual items may be of value to bookkeepers or statisticians, but it usually makes a poor impression on the patient. He or she doesn't recognize the items, wonders if he or she really received the services charged, or resents the substantial charge for an aspirin or Tylenol tablet that costs significantly less when purchased in a drugstore. These bills seem even more superfluous when one considers that most hospitals receive a flat per-diem or per-case reimbursement from third-party payers anyway.

REGIONAL AND FEDERAL HOSPITAL PLANNING

One of the first organized efforts to improve hospitals' efficiency and economy of operations was through hospital associations which incorporated planning. These efforts were limited at first to local or regional hospital organizations, and, of course, everything was done on a voluntary basis. I first became aware of regional planning in Rochester. A number of voluntary hospital associations had been developed, primarily to present a united front when mutual interests were at stake, but also to exchange information and to assist the member institutions in planning individual programs. I was particularly impressed with the Cleveland Hospital Council, the Rochester Hospital Council, and similar organizations in Pittsburgh, Philadelphia, New York City, and later Chicago and the San Francisco Bay area. With rare exceptions, these organizations concerned themselves primarily with the problems, programs, operations, and representation of the acute-care hospitals. Planning involving the overall health care system was rudimentary.

The Hill-Burton program of 1946 was the first to set and enforce national standards of hospital construction. I served on the Hill-Burton Federal Hospital Council from 1951 to 1958, and I enjoyed every session, not only because of the caliber of the members and our unique authority, but because of our accomplishments. Marshall Schaffer, the chief architect for the program, and his associates established standards for corridors, rooms, doors, fire protection, exits, and basic construction. These regulations—developed and administered at the federal level by competent professionals and enforced through licensing and funding—proved immensely helpful to hospital administrators throughout the nation. Many of the requirements developed are in force today.

The Hill-Burton program unfortunately suffered from a problem that I have observed plaguing federal programs for almost forty years: the federal guidelines, objectives, and standards were fine, but local interpretation and administration varied widely. The architectural standards were generally accepted—they had to be or no federal funds would be granted. But programmatic problems developed, depending on the caliber of the local staff and the local political pressure. Some states used Hill-Burton funds to construct and expand their state university medical centers. Others spent most of the money constructing small rural hospitals because of a shortage of hospital beds in rural areas. Many of these rural hospitals proved difficult to staff; on the other hand, some enabled the community to attract needed physicians.

Connecticut presented a different type of situation. The Department of Health was frankly disinterested in the Hill-Burton philosophy and program, partly because this wealthy and relatively small state had only a small Hill-Burton grant to allocate each year, and the commissioner of health did not want to have to choose among potential grant recipients. A frank effort was made to divide the available funds among all the hospitals that applied and were even remotely eligible. New York's allocation system stood in contrast to Connecticut's. In New York, John Bourke was responsible for Hill-Burton allocations. He and his staff not only carefully examined the requests from all over the state, but also tried to apply regional planning that carefully considered hospital beds as well as construction standards.

Another contribution of the Hill-Burton program has not been particularly appreciated. I was on the Federal Hospital Council when the suggestion was first made that specific funds be allotted for research relating to hospitals. The proposal excited me. I had always envied the British their Nuffield Foundation, which made many millions of pounds available for institutional and management research in health institutions. The United States had nothing even remotely comparable—probably because research in hospital function and design or anything that might involve associated health institutions had little sex appeal in comparison to virtually any project involving illness. When the Hill-Burton Advisory Council approved the allocation of some three million dollars a year for research in the mid-1950s, one of the first requests received, to no one's surprise, was from the Yale Department of Public Health's division of hospital administration, which proposed to study hospital function and design. Yale got its grant and recruited John Thompson, who introduced a statistical, analytical approach to hospital research, the use of the queuing theory, and field analyses of population, usages, and needs as contrasted to earlier rule-of-thumb hospital standards. I believe that his and Robert Fetter's DRG concept, which was born in the Connecticut Regional Medical Program in the late 1960s, is a legitimate offspring of that original Hill-Burton grant.

In the 1950s, the Federal Hospital Council also approved substantial Hill-Burton grants for a study of health needs in Puerto Rico. This was one of the first attempts to look at the health needs of a region as contrasted to its local physical and institutional needs. It is unfortunate that similar studies have not been made of other underserved regions of our country. One program which did so with remarkable accomplishments is the Indian Health Services, once it became part of the Public Health Service responsible for the Native Americans. This program has the unfortunate distinction of being largely ignored and now underfunded. There is little understanding of its accomplishments and of the methods health professionals have used to realize great advances in the health of a section of our population that has been so shamefully neglected for years. The program deserves an in-depth, professional, social, and political review.

Medicare and Medicaid were not the only federal health programs enacted in 1965–66. Health planning was to be part of the legislation, and Regional Medical Programs (RMPs) and the Comprehensive Health Planning Agencies (CHPs) were the first of many such efforts. The two organizations differed substantially in method of operation. The Regional

Medical Programs were local entities with local governing boards, and related to local medical schools, but responsible to a Washington office. The Comprehensive Health Planning Agency functioned on the level of the state. Regional subdivisions acted under federal guidelines, but the states had primary responsibility for the program. I was intimately involved with both the RMP and the CHP in both Connecticut and Illinois. My experiences with these programs were rewarding, constructive, educational, and discouraging. These episodes, plus later work in Connecticut with the Health Systems Agency Program of 1974 made up additional courses in my post-graduate education in government and bureaucracy.

As soon as the RMP legislation was passed, Richard Weinerman and Robert Lawton, of the Yale Medical School Dean's Office, John Thompson, and I started planning for a Connecticut RMP. We included representatives from the newly formed University of Connecticut Medical School and persuaded the commissioner of health to assume a leadership role and to appoint formally the representatives of Yale and the University of Connecticut to draw up the program and present the application. Harvard wanted to be the center of an overall New England RMP, but we politely spurned these advances and formally presented a separate application for Connecticut. The Connecticut RMP was one of the first five RMPs approved by Washington. By the fall of 1966, it was in full organizational swing. In many ways, our early formation and organization was good. Because we were new, few restricting ground rules had been developed in Washington, and by the time such rules were established Connecticut had momentum that the Washington bureau couldn't derail.

The Connecticut RMP developed a close working relationship with lay and business leaders, with the two medical schools, and with the leaders of the hospital and medical professions. It also involved organized medicine, the hospital organizations, and the state health and mental health commissioners. It took a broad view of its mission: while the federal act called for the RMPs to focus on "heart, stroke and cancer and related diseases," the CRMP wanted to strengthen all the components of teaching, diagnosis, and treatment of disease, believing this the best way to improve treatment of those specific diseases. Thus it regarded the entire health system as within its province. This meant support of both hospitals and physicians, and the various other health components as well. The Connecticut program encouraged appointment of full-time chiefs of service in the acute-care hospitals with remarkable success (see chapter 4). It also urged hospitals to affiliate with medical schools and helped hospitals obtain adequate financing and support for their teaching, research, and patient care responsibilities.

There were three unfortunate impediments to the progress of the CRMP. The first was the leaders of the state medical society, who fought RMP every inch of the way—not only in Connecticut, but also in Washington. Throughout the life of the CRMP, the Connecticut State Medical Society was a suspicious opponent. This unfortunate and puzzling attitude remained despite every effort to work with organized medicine in Connecticut by involving many medical leaders in the hospitals, the specialties, and the state medical society. There was genuine and constructive support from many prominent physicians, but this did not silence the fears of the medical society.

The second unfortunate problem involved the Connecticut Comprehensive Health Planning program (CCHP). Because Connecticut's was one of the first five RMPs in the country and because its leaders took a very broad view of their assignment, when the CCHP finally started work it found that the CRMP had already assumed a great deal of responsibility that the CCHP believed was within its province. This, along with the organizational problems of the national Comprehensive Health Planning Program and the relative lack of interest of the Connecticut State Department of Health—which was politically responsible for the CCHP, but whose commissioner evinced more interest in the CRMP—left the CCHP agencies floundering for both program and mission.

Finally, the CRMP became the victim of the same malady of changing federal leadership, directives, and emphasis that cripples so many federal-state programs. The contradictory signals from the federal office made it difficult for the state organization to present a coherent program to its constituency. And so the RMP—as with the CHP and HSA—became another program for which millions of dollars were appropriated with the best of intentions, but which failed and was finally abandoned. In addition to the massive financial expenditures, citizens gave thousands of hours to these programs that were then abandoned in favor of another alternative, also destined to be short-lived.

An unfortunate side effect of the federal government's abortive involvement with health planning was the abolition of many voluntary health and hospital planning agencies. These casualties resulted from lack of financing or from deliberate efforts by CHPs and HSAs to eliminate such organizations, which were considered antagonistic, competitive, or unnecessary. The CHPC, the Bay Area Health Facilities Planning Association, the Hospital Planning Council of Metropolitan Chicago—all fell victims. Voluntary planning agencies in Detroit, Pittsburgh, and, to an extent, New York City survived. Many people honestly believed that the voluntary programs were unnecessary because the government agencies would have the stature, funds, and authority to make their voluntary counterparts superfluous. The tragedy, of course, was that the government agencies were then, one after another, eliminated by Washington.

Although planning would seem to be a logical component of any systematic approach to the delivery of health care and the containment of costs, it was soon found to be ineffective by itself. Health costs showed no evidence of doing anything but increasing. Part of this was because the system of regional, state, and federal health planning had no real authority and had been tinkered with to the point of confusion, emasculation, or destruction.

REGULATION AND CONTROL OF HOSPITALS

The rapidly increasing costs of health care, not only for individuals, but also for third-party payers, stimulated the creation of authoritative regulation and control methods to contain cost. This has presented a different set of problems to the hospital and its CEO. Now he or she must face the problem of adapting the hospital's own planning to a variety of ever-changing fiscal restraints. In addition, departments that were once concerned only with rate structure and reimbursement have now become deeply involved in the planning for construction, major equipment, and even programs and services. Hospital and health administrators have been forced to make radical adjustments far beyond the early construction standards. The constructive advances that came out of the 1946 Hill-Burton program conditioned me to believe in the value of standards, regulations, and controls. Neither Dr. MacLean nor I had any illusions about the effectiveness of self-regulation—either by the individual institution or that institution's local or state organization—where costs are concerned. But, although I accept the fact that it is appropriate for state or federal government to develop control mechanisms, the problem is, Who? Over what? and How?

In the early 1950s, cost control was only a theoretical possibility. It was not even much of a concern to me in the early 1960s, although I wondered what might happen when third parties reimbursed hospitals for a high percentage of their patients. Ray Brown of Chicago was one of the first hospital leaders to recognize the dangers of the extraordinarily rapid hospital cost increases. But my efforts toward state hospital planning had little to do with health costs. I was primarily concerned to develop a sensible plan for acute-care hospital facilities throughout the state. I assumed that reason would prevail. However, a short time after I had begun my efforts, a small hospital in a neighboring town received a gift of several hundred thousand dollars to construct a twenty-bed maternity unit. Two larger hospitals in the town had empty obstetric beds. No one, except the donor, the small hospital, and a few of its medical staff, could see the slightest reason for the additional unit. The CHPC, the state commissioner of health, the Hill-Burton program, and almost everyone else strongly disapproved. But the hospital had the money, the medical staff and board supported the plan, and the unit was built. I remember predicting that if the hospital went ahead in spite of all this advice and pressure, the state would probably develop some sort of restrictive licensing or control mechanism for construction of health facilities. My prediction was correct: from the 1965 infusion of federal Medicare money and the associated sprouting of federal-state planning and development agencies emerged the new concept of Certificate of Need (CON). This usually took the form of an official body (usually in the state government) which would issue a formal approval or permit theoretically based upon demonstrated need for major capital expenditures for construction or equipment.

At first I thought that CON would only make sure that too many hospital beds would not be constructed. But by the time the various federal planning programs were put into effect, health costs were continuing to rise, and regulations and control on programs, costs, and reimbursement seemed logical and inevitable. The obvious target remained the hospital. I used the hospital's vulnerability myself when I worked for the governor of Illinois. Health costs were mounting rapidly. We recognized the role of the physicians, but there were several thousand physicians and dentists in Illinois, and only about 250 hospitals. Most of the health care money was being paid to hospitals, so they were the logical points of attack. We hoped that they would pass this pressure to reduce costs on to the medical staff, but this turned out to be wishful thinking. Even where state CON legislation was enacted, community or political pressure, along with the provider's influence and persistence, usually meant that the applicant eventually got most of the money requested—and the delay merely made the project more expensive.

My experience in Illinois was, overall, a delightful one. But my work with regulations and control on health institutions and health costs proved discouraging and puzzling. I found a strong and respected hospital association and able and competent hospital leaders, all interested in high quality patient care and in efficiency and economy. However, as I sat across the table from them in my position as coordinator for health services in the Office of the Governor, I was amused to find that the hospital administrators made the same arguments and took the same positions as I had when I was the CEO of Yale-New Haven. Many of their arguments seemed as specious and self-serving as had been many of mine. They, quite understandably, looked first to the welfare of their own institutions.

The hospital is such an essential component of our health delivery system that every effort must be made to strengthen and support it. Yet, as health costs continue to rise and alternatives are developed for some traditional hospital functions, adjustments must be made. Cost-based payment for services; restrictions on expansion in size, service, or equipment; and more efficient combinations or use of facilities are only a few of the elements essential to lowering costs in the overall health system. Voluntary associations, consortia, and planning were a beginning, but they are insufficient as costs and health care facilities burgeon—and goals other than simply improving health care for more people appear. Certificate of Need legislation was of some value, but only when staff were competent to make intelligent and equitable recommendations to the decision-making body. Experience and professional impartiality are essential. With all its complications and potential limitations, the DRG approach has had the greatest impact on hospital costs and utilization. It remains to be seen what else is needed.

STATE RATE COMMISSIONS

The next major development in cost control was the creation of state rate commissions for hospitals. Most functioned through a combination of budget and rate control, along with various CON arrangements for approving construction, programs, and equipment. The statewide bodies, mostly in the eastern states, the DRG prospective pricing system for Medicare, and the efforts to extend this approach to all payers are the latest developments in regulation and control for the health delivery system.

I can look at these developments with relative detachment, for it is my students and former associates, not I, who must live with them. I don't know that I fully agree with the comment that I lived in the Golden Age of hospital administration, nor am I yet prepared to believe that "hospital administration is no fun anymore." But the present climate of regulation and control can be frustrating and worrisome. The state rate commissions provide an excellent example of the problems associated with government regulation. When I helped develop the legislation for the Connecticut Hospital Cost Commission in 1949–50, our hospital per-diem costs were approximately ten dollars a day, and the commission's primary responsibility was to assure that these costs were accurately calculated. In 1973,

the Connecticut Commission on Hospitals and Health Care was established. The legislature gave the commission broad authority over hospital
rates, budgets, major changes in programs and services, and major
purchases in equipment. The commission could and did exert strong
control over the administration and operations of Connecticut acute-care
hospitals.

After an initial legal confrontation, for about three years hospitals
had enjoyed relatively amicable, constructive relations with the commission. This abruptly changed when the governor appointed a new
executive officer. Although the legislative mandate and the commission's
membership remained essentially unchanged, relations between the
Commission and the hospitals changed markedly. An epidemic of court
actions took place. From 1976 through 1983, Connecticut hospitals
mounted more than forty legal challenges to the commission's actions,
and the vast majority of the decisions were won by the hospitals.

As a result of this turmoil, the Connecticut legislature altered the
makeup of the commission in 1981 from a group of seventeen part-time,
voluntary members to a full-time commission of three. The governor
appointed the former executive director as chairman. More lawsuits
occurred, most of which were again decided in favor of the hospitals. The
problems continued until a new chairman and executive officer were
appointed in 1983. Working relationships between the controlling agency
and the hospitals then improved substantially, primarily because of the
new executive officer's different personality and approach to his responsibilities. I had the opportunity to discuss with the former director his
program and objectives. He was well-informed, determined, sure of
himself, and impatient. I could not argue with his overall objectives. But
with the growing complexity of the health service industry and the
immense amount of money and special interests involved, an individual
or a group with an impatient bureaucratic or autocratic approach, even
with the best of intentions, will find themselves forever fighting with the
providers— particularly when money or survival is involved. Resentment is further aroused when only hospitals are regulated and private
physicians are immune. Regulation of private physicians is only beginning to be explored.

Authority should be commensurate with responsibility, especially in
a regulatory body. As already pointed out, the Connecticut commission
can exert great control over hospital administration and operation. But it is
the hospitals that are ultimately responsible for the care of patients. This
separation of authority and responsibility is a dangerous situation which
can only be defused by competent, professional leadership in the reg-

ulatory body and smooth and constructive lines of communication between the commission and health institutions. Because of their direct influence on costs and on patient care, physicians cannot remain uninvolved, even though many will find distasteful the concept of review of their orders and actions.

DEFINING GOALS AND POLICIES

A major shortcoming that underlies our attempts to improve the delivery of health care is the lack of a clearly defined national policy or goal. This deficiency seems to contribute to virtually every difficulty discussed in this book. The creation of such goals is a major challenge to the health care system, the government, and society at large. Once they are defined, we can turn to the complicating factors of developing logical methods to attain them and of measuring our progress toward their attainment.

The problem of what the mechanism of control or the nature of the controlling body should be has continued to escape solution. The responsibility of federal or state governments, or both, has been advocated. Those delivering health services, industry—which pays a substantial part of the costs, and the customer (the patient), also believe that government should be involved. I agree. I have never hesitated to call upon government to finance the health care of those who cannot pay for themselves. I never saw anything wrong with government playing a major role in a health care control system—not only because I knew that the private health system would not (or could not) control its own complex organization, but also because government will continue to underwrite a high percentage of the cost. The federal and state share of spending for health care may now be over 40 percent. Also, as I have stated, social forces are so closely allied to health that some overall influence is needed. Government certainly figures in such a role. When we add industry's financial stake in health care, we begin to understand the complexity of the forces involved in the effort to control the health care industry. The simplest approach to cost control is regulation based upon formulae that range from simplistic and rigid to those subject to a bewildering array of variations and adjustments. Government is the most logical body to authorize and enforce cost-control formulae, providing it has a sensible policy, competent staff, and a constructive liaison with all affected parties.

Industry is a relative latecomer to the problems of health care control. I recall with appreciation the support of Eastman Kodak and other companies in Rochester in the 1940s for the principle of community rating and the Rochester Blue Cross plan. And the support from industrial leaders in

Connecticut over the years has been crucial in maintaining the strength of Connecticut hospitals and their association. But, in general, industry often reminds me of the old Southern mule that one had to hit on the head with a two-by-four to get its attention. I tried in 1976 and 1981 to get the Connecticut leaders in medicine, hospitals, labor, the bureaucracy, education, and business together to look at the Connecticut health system as a whole.[4] I met with little interest or understanding. But today, the dollar is the two-by-four that is getting industry's attention. The Chrysler Corporation and Joseph Califano, Jr., are excellent examples.

The next set of problems confronting those concerned with regulation and control of the health system include its organization, administration, and leadership at the federal, state, and local levels. I have learned that, at the state and regional level, not only the senior personnel but the competence of the entire staff is vital—particularly in the agencies responsible for licensure, regulation, and control. Today, the CEO of a major hospital and his or her staff may spend weeks planning programs, services, and budgets. Although the CEO has final responsibility to the board, the medical staff, the community, and the patients regarding the type, quality, and cost of the services provided by the hospital, the bureaucracy may have the last word on what can be done and what will be paid for. As mentioned earlier, the problems involved in the separation of authority and responsibility are starkly clear.

For example, in 1984, the Maine Health Care Finance Commission froze hospital programs, refusing to accept anything that did not appear in 1983 budgets. The rigidity of the system requires an inordinate amount of effort and circumlocution to accomplish the obvious. One hospital was forbidden to employ a radiologist on salary because in 1983 the radiologist was paid by the fee-for-service system. When we were fighting our battles with the American College of Radiology and the AMA over salary thirty years ago, I never dreamed that the state bureaucracy would be our next opponents!

The governing board of the hospital and its CEO have legal and moral responsibility for the welfare of the hospital's patients. The physician has responsibility for his or her own patients. The health care corporation or institution is responsible for the health and welfare of the community in which it exists. None of these responsibilities can be blithely ignored. But those who bear them must function within bounds, restrictions, or controls that are established by some other body, which may exercise its authority through prohibition, restriction, or refusal of funds. Profession-

4. A. Snoke and P. Snoke, "Linking Private, Public Energies in Health and Welfare Planning," *Hospitals* 16, 16 (August 16, 1976), 53–58.

als, not amateurs or politicians, must be the ones exercising this authority. Unfortunately, it is not easy to define what makes a "professional" in this specific situation.

THE CONSUMER AND COMPETITION

I am made increasingly uncomfortable by the expectation that the influence of the marketplace—advertising, marketing, competition, options, deductibles, and co-insurance—will result in wise decisions by the customer, the patient, or the family. These terms, plus the growing interest of government and industry in health costs, have prompted John Inglehart to ask whether these payers consider medical care an economic product or a social goal.[5] Certainly, the simplistic idea that competition is an effective or rational mechanism for cost containment is not particularly realistic if the buyer must make judgments on quality. This is especially true of patients. They have so little knowledge upon which to base intelligent choices when they are confronted with competitive offers or opportunities. Because of my years of working with other health professionals, I am in a far better position than most lay individuals to make judgments regarding medication, treatments, and specialists. But I have no illusions—I don't know modern medicine, nor do 99 percent of those obtaining advice and care, and I and they must depend upon the advice and judgment of a trusted physician. I may be in a better position to select that individual, but having done so I must rely on his or her judgment, not upon the competitive offer.

The individual cannot plan for his or her future care on the basis of competition any more than that person or his or her family, when confronted with an emergency, will automatically be prudent buyers because of the existence of co-insurance and deductibles. I have yet to see family members debate costs in the emergency room of the hospital admitting office when someone is brought in acutely ill. The family almost invariably wants whatever the hospital or the attending physician considers necessary.

Our traditional health system and traditional methods of payment haven't really helped patients and families make cost-conscious decisions. But progress is slowly being made. I have worked with men and women who helped develop improved organization for the provision and financing of health care. I think they would agree that the individual and family are at a disadvantage when they are expected to make an informed

5. J. K. Inglehart, "Fixed-Fee Medicine for Medicare: An Introduction to Prospective Payment," *Issues in Science and Technology* (Fall 1984), 95–100.

choice in health matters on the basis of competition or aggressive marketing. They need a mechanism upon which they can depend, by which they can obtain competent fiscal and professional advice on health care.

These are excellent arguments for the development of patient-care organizations dedicated to the philosophy of a continuum of care through a vertical integration of facilities and resources. Such a program could be financed on a prepayment, group practice, or HMO basis. It would also have available expertise necessary to evaluate quality and service, so as to protect patients and families from greedy entrepreneurs. With the increasing formation of national supercorporations, sophisticated patient-oriented organizations and competent government control mechanisms will become even more necessary. I hope competition as advocated by Enthoven and Noll can then exist and be fair to those needing health care.

This would merely be a formalization of my repeated efforts to put the right patient in the right place at the right time with a minimum of expense and red tape. It is now being tried in Greenville, South Carolina. The Greenville Hospital System, with some nine institutional units, has expanded its horizons to the aspects of health care outside the institutional walls. Home health care, "Lifeline," ambulatory care facilities, and hospice are all part of the continuum of care philosophy even though they are hesitant to identify themselves as a Greenville Health System.

If we add prepayment and HMO-type financing to this administrative and corporate organization, individuals or families would not be directly confronted by competition, salesmanship, and marketing. They could turn to organizations for professional judgment and advice, as well as cost-conscious health care. As with any organization, its policies and goals, performance record, the character and concern of its governing board, and the competence, experience, and probity of the chief executive officer will be crucial measures of its success.

We do not yet know enough to advocate any specific system or even a limited number of alternate systems. Our present fee-for-service system presents problems when multiple procedures are more profitable to the physician than spending the same amount of time trying to understand and reassure the patients through personal contact. But this can be corrected.

I hope that those who pay for health care will continue to support service organizations that consider health a right, not a privilege. But we also need to recognize that the complexity and the enormity of these organizations providing care will still require some regulation and control. I also hope that such analysis and control will be carried out by professionals under clear policies developed by society at large and that our ultimate concern will be the proper care of all people.

9

Government and Health

Government's current massive involvement in health is really a development of the past half century. The federal government's health activities began with the U.S. Public Health Service (USPHS). It first focused on communicable disease, quarantine regulations, and its long-established responsibility for the health of the merchant seamen. By the 1940s, health care for veterans began to assume greater importance, but these programs were still second-rate at best—"old soldiers' homes" were the familiar local evidence of this federal responsibility. State and local departments of health dealt chiefly with environmental protection, communicable disease, and vital statistics.

Although I became acquainted with the USPHS during World War II, I did not learn much about health planning for the country as a whole until the late 1950s. The Hoover Commissions on the responsibilities of federal health programs, Martha Eliot and the federal Children's Bureau, and the earlier Emergency Maternal and Infant Care program (EMIC) were important national health activities, but they dealt with specific issues. I was exposed to the shift in thinking, planning, and authority of the national health power structure through my membership in 1947 in the Society of Medical Administrators (SMA), which is made up of many of the physician leaders in hospital and health care administration. During the 1940s and 1950s, I learned of problems, programs, and developments in national health from the senior members of the SMA. Many of them played active roles in influencing the course of national health planning.

By 1960, this had changed. Plans and developments were being decided upon by government, not by associates, unless they happened to be part of the federal establishment. This fundamental shift in power was the subject of my 1965 speech upon accepting the AHA's Distinguished

Service Award. It was never published by the AHA journal, *Hospitals*, and I was never sure whether because of the subject, the length—or a decision that "elder statesmen" should be seen and decorated but not read. The speech was certainly neither polite nor diplomatic for 1965. I praised the medical profession's accomplishments but criticized their organization and their leaders, as well as my hospital colleagues, for failing to implement professional and scientific advances in the care of people. I emphasized the importance of that amorphous group called "the public"—they were paying the bill, I said, and should be considered partners. I reminded my audience that the public was looking to us for guidance, and that if we did not respond constructively they would make their decisions without us. I decried the inability of the two great health organizations, AMA and AHA, to work together constructively to advise Congress on Medicare, the most important health legislation yet enacted. And I criticized all of us for not being willing to explore improved systems for the delivery of health care. I was also critical of our voluntary institutions (hospitals, medical staffs, and universities) and the government health establishment for not recognizing the expertise of individuals who were trained to meet the changing demands of health administration.

This speech described what I had observed and learned, since 1940, from the leaders of the voluntary health system and from the PHS professionals. From 1940 to 1980, I was closely associated with the people in federal health, particularly in the USPHS, and came to respect that division and many of its members tremendously. I would have joined many of my friends who received commissions in the USPHS under George Baehr in 1941—but when I had received my appointment and told Dr. MacLean that I was being measured for my uniform, he said that he outranked me as a lieutenant colonel in the office of the Surgeon General of the Army (which he had joined as a consultant) and that I was to stay home as acting director of Strong Memorial Hospital. I did, but I became acquainted with many commissioned officers in the PHS and learned what might be accomplished through competent, professional leadership at the national level. From working with them I became convinced of the vital importance of recruiting, developing, utilizing, and *retaining* the best of professional health leadership in government as well as in the private sector.

My experience with the federal government came not only through my friendship with USPHS officers but also from serving on advisory boards for a number of its divisions and other sections of the federal establishment concerned with health, such as the Department of Defense and the Veterans Administration. My closest friend from 1939 until his death in 1969 was Jack Masur. He became a PHS commissioned officer in

1942. While in Rochester I worked with him in the planning of the National Institutes of Health Clinical Center at Bethesda. We spent hours trying to adjust reality to the requirements and expectations of the many clinical and preclinical scientists who expected to use the hospital facilities. I don't believe there is a professor or research scientist in existence who does not have an exaggerated (but perfectly logical to him or her) concept of the space and equipment required for his or her particular specialty. Part of Dr. Masur's responsibility in the PHS was the Hill-Burton Program. As a member of the Federal Hospital Council, I went to Washington frequently and usually ended up—via several secretaries and a private elevator—in his spacious office. During one of my visits, a subordinate was ushered in on appointment because of some failure in judgment or performance. Dr. Masur, whom I thought the gentlest and most considerate of people, tonguelashed his subordinate and dismissed him with the dire threat that if he did not improve he would be appointed quarantine officer of the Pribiloff Islands off Alaska— inhabited primarily by seals. After the individual had slunk away I remarked that senior officers in the Public Health Service must get tired of a diet of raw meat. Dr. Masur stared at me silently for a long time and then remarked that one of the most difficult problems he faced in military and government service was in realizing the awesome power senior officials had over subordinates. How easy it was to forget to be human or fair! I have tried never to forget that episode and Dr. Masur's obvious embarrassment at his lapse.

During those years, when I worked closely with Masur and other members of the Commissioned Officer Corps of the PHS, I came to respect them, the Surgeon Generals, and later the Assistant Secretaries for Health Affairs. They were all health professionals and did not hesitate to discuss frankly their hopes, policies, and programs for people's health. Thus I was particularly impressed during the early 1950s with their nervousness and obvious discomfort with the subject of Senator Joseph McCarthy. The reactions of these superior professionals to this type of politician made a lasting impression upon me. I can only compare the supportive contributions of individuals like Senator Lister Hill and Representative John Fogarty with the almost malignant influence of Senator McCarthy and hope that the voters and those in government will be vigilant in opposing the ascendency of another such individual in the future, as well as weeding out the vestiges of his ideology that are still alive today.

PHS AND THE BUREAU OF THE BUDGET

In early 1956 I was introduced to a phenomenon that confronts all operating officers but is seemingly intensified in government: the authority of the budget officer. I had gone to Washington to attend a meeting of the Advisory Committee of the Servicemen's Dependent's Program (then still called Medicare), and Deputy Surgeon General W. Palmer Dearing asked me to lunch. The PHS ran a number of hospitals throughout the country and was having great difficulty obtaining sufficient funds for their operation. Fred McNamara in the Bureau of the Budget had assumed direct responsibility for the PHS hospital budget—and although costs and wages were mounting, appropriations were being cut back.

From our discussion, we developed a consultation program, the strategy of which was mapped out on paper doilies. We first accepted the fact that long-range decisions about the PHS hospital program were a matter of national policy and should be made by political bodies, not by the Bureau of the Budget. This question has now been settled with the abolition of the program, but at that time, the institutions were considered to be performing a useful function. The hospitals were scattered all over the country, and Dr. Dearing did not have the funds for a major consulting project. But I suggested that in every PHS hospital location we knew senior administrators that were respected hospital leaders. So the paper doilies listed the name and location of each hospital and the local hospital leader, whom I would tap for review. We chose G. Otis Whitecotton in San Francisco, Frank Bradley in St. Louis, Ray Brown in Chicago, and Josh McIntyre in New Orleans, and I chose the Staten Island Hospital for my own review.

All the consultants accepted, and my wife and I went down to Staten Island with my chief nurse, dietician, engineer, purchasing agent, controller, head nurse, chief surgical resident, and chief medical resident. Each individual spent two days with his or her Staten Island counterpart. Dr. Parnie and I, and an administrative associate, worked with the administrative staff. The next morning we met with all the participants to coordinate our findings. By the end of two days I had learned enough to prepare the report promptly. My first draft criticized the Bureau of the Budget's reductions, saying the bureau was taking off the clothes, skin, and the muscles and closely approaching the bone. My wife suggested that I call this an exaggeration of the ecdysiastical approach. I said, "What in hell is *ecdysiastical*?" She patiently explained that H. L. Mencken had coined the term *ecdysiast*—meaning stripteaser—in 1925, and Walter Winchell had picked it up in his newspaper column. I thought this was wonderful and incorporated the term in my report.

All the reports were sent to Dr. Dearing and, some weeks later, I was asked to come to Washington to discuss the reports with the new surgeon general, Leroy Burney. He greeted me with courtesy, thanked me for giving him ammunition to counteract the influence of the Bureau of the

Budget, and asked me only one question: what was the ecdysiastical approach? I was pleased to learn that appropriations for the PHS hospitals would now be realistic.

PUBLIC HEALTH LEADERSHIP AND ORGANIZATION

The health labor force and health leadership were two items that preoccupied me and many PHS leaders, especially Jack Masur, as we worked together on the many projects, advisory boards, and experimental activities involving the government and private sector. I was impressed with the custom whereby PHS personnel were lent to states as directors of health (Leroy Burney went to Indiana, Herman Hilleboe to New York). Because of this interest in career development, I did not understand why the federal government later allowed its health professionals to deteriorate. I wrote of this in a 1969 article for the *American Journal of Public Health*.[1] I was flattered when Myron Wegman, dean of the University of Michigan School of Public Health, discussed my theme in his 1962 presidential address to the APHA.[2]

In 1937, PHS officers and the surgeon generals were highly respected health professionals. But deterioration of the Commissioned Officer Corps of the PHS and the emasculation of the office of Surgeon General started in the early 1960s, along with an extensive series of reorganizations.[3]

For a number of compelling reasons it seemed appropriate to examine the organization and leadership of the USPHS in the late 1950s and early 1960s. By then, an increased sense of social responsibility had put health issues high on the agenda in the eyes of the public, Congress, and health leaders. Although some individual PHS members did provide leadership

1. A. Snoke, "The Unsolved Problems of the Career Professional in the Establishment of National Health Policy," *AJPH* 59 (1969), 1575–88.

2. M. E. Wegman, "Centennial Presidential Address (American Public Health Association): Policy, Priority, and the Power to Act," *AJPH* 63, 2 (1973), 98–101.

3. I found in my experience with state governments that reorganization can be a major handicap to efficiency and economy and particularly to retaining competent personnel. Unfortunately, this is not a modern phenomenon. The following quotation was attributed to Petronius Arbiter in Nero's court in 66 A.D.: "We trained hard, but it seemed that every time we were beginning to form into teams, we would be reorganized. I was to learn later in life that we tend to meet a new situation by reorganizing, and a wonderful method it can be for creating the illusion of progress, while producing confusion, inefficiency, and demoralization." This was repeated by Professor Lawrence of *The Peter Principle* fame in his 1977 book of *Peter's Quotations*. Neither Professor Lawrence, the Yale Rare Book Library, Petronius' *Satyricon*, nor I have been able to come up with the original. I now suspect that some disillusioned person invented the quotation and attributed it to Petronius. Notwithstanding its origin, it is appropriate not only to 66 A.D. but to the 1980s.

in these areas, neither the PHS nor its career officers in general appeared committed to solving the problem of providing health care for the public. This was partly due to opposition by the AMA and its regional components to PHS officers' becoming involved in the provision of medical care. The PHS commissioned officers also suffered because a growing number of federal civil servants in other health programs resented them as a relatively small, "elite" group that appeared to favor those who had come up through the traditional PHS Commissioned Corps ranks.

Whatever the reasons, there was substantial dissatisfaction in the late 1950s and early 1960s with the Commissioned Corps of the PHS. They seemed unwilling or unable to face modern problems related to administration and delivery of health service. The status of the Commissioned Corps did not improve during the long battle over Medicare, for many members remained aloof until the new program was about to be passed.

As the numbers of dollars, people, and programs involved with health care increased over the years, the PHS, with its limited number of career personnel and its traditional orientation, was overwhelmed and bypassed by other federal health programs, developed outside of HEW, as well as programmed outside the PHS itself. The resultant competition for personnel, funds, and authority resulted in seemingly endless reorganization in HEW and the PHS.

Congressman John Fogarty (who, unlike Senator Lister Hill, was never recognized for his contributions to health) stimulated reorganization planning for PHS around 1959–60. It is not generally realized that this 1960 report and its philosophy came from a committee and staff made up primarily of Commissioned Corps leaders of the PHS—the same group that had been accused of being reactionary, conservative, or nonperceptive. This report resulted in a number of administrative and organizational changes in PHS, and stimulated John Gardner, secretary of HEW, to commission another reorganization study in 1966 under the direction of John J. Corson and a committee drawn from outside the department. This was one of the major milestones in changing the philosophy and structure of the PHS. It was no longer built around a professional staff and headed by a professional careerperson with statutory invulnerability, but an organization much more influenced by changing personalities and partisan politics.

In addition to the 1966 reorganization, which reshuffled the bureaus and services within the PHS, the authority of the Office of the Surgeon General was substantially weakened. The surgeon general was not given line control over programs, budget, or staff. The position evolved into that of a staff officer to the assistant secretary for health and scientific affairs, a newly created political position. This began to develop with the 1961 appointment of Boisfeuillet Jones as special assistant for health and medical affairs, followed in 1964–65 by Edward Dempsey, dean of the Medical School at Washington University at St. Louis. Philip Lee then assumed responsibility in a more authoritative position as assistant secretary for health and scientific affairs. William Stewart was surgeon general of the PHS during this time, and he assisted in the emasculation—expecting that he would be the last surgeon general of the PHS.

Before the 1966 reorganization was made official, Secretary Gardner announced his intention for further changes in the PHS. The new plan, which went into effect in the spring of 1968, under the direction of Acting Secretary Wilbur Cohen, was the product of a second Corson committee. It created three administrations: research and education (NIH), health services (Health Services and Mental Health Administration), and consumer and environmental health activities (Consumer Protection and Environmental Health Services). All reported directly to the assistant secretary for health and scientific affairs, Dr. Lee, who was responsible for the health programs of HEW. Further recommendations were made by Secretary Cohen in June. One was that a position of deputy secretary for health be approved by Congress. As a result, the assistant secretary for health and scientific affairs became directly responsible to the secretary of HEW for the health programs within the purview of the PHS. Thus, the surgeon general became a staff officer with virtually no supporting staff and no direct operating authority.

I have never tried to belittle the role of the assistant secretary of health and scientific affairs. Those officers have been of value to the health world. They have without exception been persons of stature and ability, selected because of their preeminence in their particular fields. I have been proud that many of them were friends of mine. But I am critical of their organizational background and particularly the length of stay in this important and prestigious position, which has averaged less than three years.

The secretaryship of HEW (now HHS) is traditionally held for an average of two years. This is understandable for a political position. But when this phenomenon also occurs in the office of assistant secretary, and when one reflects that upon the importance of the federal government's responsibility for the health and welfare of the people, the vast number of personnel involved, and the billions of dollars spent annually, a crucial question comes up. I first raised it in 1969, and repeated it in 1983: "What has happened to the rest of the professional leadership for health in the federal government, from the surgeon general on down?"[4] The same

4. A. Snoke, "What Good is Legislation—or Planning—If We Can't Make It Work? The Need for a Comprehensive Approach to Health and Welfare," *AJPH* 72, 9 (1982), 1028–33.

question must be directed at the stability and priorities of the organization. The keen interest in cost containment has unfortunately resulted in a shift in influence over health planning from health professionals to fiscal officers and budget directors at both the state and federal levels. A public memorandum by Charles C. Edwards, who resigned as assistant secretary for health in January, 1975, outlined the frustration of one health professional in dealing with the system:

The method used in determining the figures totally undermines our efforts to manage the health agencies.... OMB (Office of Management and Budget) has removed necessary management flexibility, separated accountability from authority, and destroyed the entire planning and budgeting system we spent years building.... If these actions truly represent the administration's philosophy, we may as well have six health agencies reporting directly to the OMB.[5]

The budget director and the Office of Management and Budget are rightly concerned about the billions of dollars spent for health and welfare. Blank checks should not be issued in the name of health and welfare any more than they should be issued in the name of defense. But I plead for stability of organization and leadership, and a rational, consistent, broad policy to help us retain leaders and staff necessary to oversee this stupendous expenditure. Who should be developing the policy, the program, and the training, assuring the continuity of leadership, and following up on this vital aspect of our national well-being? Should it be professionals, amateurs, politicians, or bureaucrats? The appointment of C. Everett Koop as surgeon general—a man with a long background in pediatric surgery, pronounced views on abortion, and so little public health experience that even the American Public Health Association felt compelled to protest his appointment—is not encouraging.

Criticisms of the revolving-door phenomenon for health leaders and the continual musical chair rearrangement of management and organization are said to be unrealistic given this country's political bureaucracy. I don't think so. Many aspects of the military or industrial corporate complexes are criticized, but a continuity of experienced leadership and retention of able professionals is generally accepted as good practice. Some may interpret frequent changes at the senior level as progress. On the other hand, this presumably constructive activity may only be Brownian Movement—rapid oscillation of minute particles suspended in certain fluids, without the slightest evidence of progress. Change is no guarantee of progress. Consider the subordinates trying to work in a

5. C. E. Edwards, Memorandum to HEW Secretary Caspar Weinberger, December, 1974; *New York Times*, February 3, 1975.

continually changing environment. One friend of mine, who served as head of a major division for twelve years, worked under four presidents, seven secretaries of HEW/HHS, eight assistant secretaries of health, three surgeon generals, and ten senior administrators! Under these circumstances, effective performance can only be happenstance. Even the experience and dedication of a superlative career civil servant can be eroded or frustrated by continually changing signals and superiors.

Accompanying this confusion in the federal administrative bureaucracy in health affairs has been the growth of the legislative bureaucracy in the same field. While the administrative bureaus were organizing or recruiting staff, congressional committees and individual members were collecting their own staffs of experts. Some, like Jay Constantine, Irving Wolkstein, and Val Halamandaris, remained for a number of years and assisted Congress in a constructive manner. Others were assigned responsibilities and given authority which they had neither the competence nor the experience to handle. These "instant experts," along with their frequently changing leaders in the administrative bureaus, are the architects of too much human services legislation. They have produced one brave new program after another, each with detailed subsections requiring voluminous regulations, each of which is finally found unworkable, thus requiring further changes or new legislation.

This is the system that described the purpose of the RMPs legislation as improvement of health care, personnel, and facilities "without interfering with the patterns, or the methods of financing, of professional care or professional practice, or with the administration of hospitals."[6] The similar legislation introducing the CHP program the following year stated again that the intent was "to assure comprehensive health services of high quality for every person, but without interference with existing patterns of private professional practice of medicine, dentistry and related healing arts."[7]

Prospective physicians receive an education designed to train them for the profession. When I became a hospital administrator, I recognized the need for education and training in that field, and I tried to provide the appropriate environment for my students. There are a number of programs that try to do the same for public health. There are schools for business, organization, and management, and any industry or business

6. Public Law 89–239. Purposes, An Act to Amend the Public Health Service Act to Assist in Combating Heart Disease, Cancer, Stroke, and Related Disease (Regional Medical Program). Congressional Act, S. 596, October 16, 1965, p. 1.

7. Public Law 89–749. Findings and Declaration of Purpose. Comprehensive Health Planning and Public Health Services Amendments of 1966. 89th Congress, November 3, 1966, p. 1.

has a definite pattern for recruitment, training, and retention of competent personnel. All are concerned with improving their organization and administration. But how is health, one of the largest industries in the country and one in which government has such responsibility, addressing its national problems of organization, administration, and leadership? The preoccupation today is with cost containment, and all our hopes are placed upon the DRGs. But this is only a different method of reimbursement. Even its most enthusiastic advocates do not believe it is a root solution to the serious problems associated with health care delivery. Where, who, and what are our resources to solve them? And what should be the political administration and personnel organization of this complicated, multi-billion-dollar industry that is so vital to the health and welfare of the people? The answers are not obvious, nor am I aware of efforts to get them.

HEALTH AND HUMAN SERVICES IN ILLINOIS

From 1969 to 1973, I worked as coordinator of health services in the Office of the Governor of Illinois. This experience was a cram course in government health administration, in which I learned both the weaknesses and the strengths and potentials of the state government's role in the care of people. This appointment was my first opportunity to work directly in the political bureaucracy, a key part of our social system which up to then had been completely foreign to me. I found myself sitting on the opposite side of the table from many of my friends and former colleagues in the voluntary health field, discussing and debating with them health care planning, reimbursement, and financing. I hope that during my stay in Illinois I contributed something to the health and welfare of its people, but I know that I got much more than I gave.

My involvement with Illinois was purely accidental. At a medical conference in January, 1968, I got into a discussion with Edwin L. Crosby, executive director of the AHA, and John D. Porterfield, III, executive director of the Joint Commission on the Accreditation of Hospitals. They were both worried about the accreditation status of the Cook County Hospital in Chicago. At that time the JCAH accredited a hospital for either one year (provisional) or three years (full). If a hospital had two successive provisional accreditations, it had to improve sufficiently prior to the third examination to obtain a full accreditation or it would lose its accreditation altogether. Both men were understandably worried because Cook County Hospital had been given two provisional accreditations, and the third accreditation visit was coming up that spring. Cook County was and is a vital hospital for many people of Chicago. It had been the teaching environment of at least five Chicago-area medical schools, and much of the professional care was given by the resident staff. If the hospital lost its accreditation, the residency programs would be disapproved, with catastrophic consequences for both the hospital and its patients. Because of the importance of this survey, Dr. Portersfield had decided to send in a team of acknowledged leaders in their respective specialties instead of the JCAH's regular surveyors. Portersfield and Crosby asked me to make the administrative review. I accepted, spent several days at the hospital, and then wrote my section of the critique. The final decision on accreditation was made by the commission.

At that time, Richard B. Ogilvie was president of the Cook County Board of Supervisors, which was responsible for the hospital. Ogilvie and his associates were quite dissatisfied with its administration, and he asked me if I would come to Chicago and be its CEO. I thanked him and said that I didn't think anyone with experience would accept the position unless he or she were very hungry. Mr. Ogilvie then asked me if I would be willing to survey the administrative aspects of the institution and frankly outline what I thought ought to be done. I said I would. As a result my wife and I spent August, 1968, virtually living in the Cook County Hospital from early in the morning until late at night. It was a remarkable experience. There were only a few hospitals like it in the country—Bellevue in New York City, the Los Angeles County Hospital, and the Charity Hospital in New Orleans. However, Cook County at that time seemed to have unique problems. The Department of Nursing was an excellent example. Although the departments of Nursing and Social Services were under a separate board and supposedly immune from political pressure on their staffs, their budgets were controlled by the Cook County Board of Supervisors. I learned at first hand how this absolute control of the purse strings could alter the actions and even the very thought processes of otherwise independent professionals.

Part of my concern was obviously the budget: how it was prepared and whether it provided for sufficient personnel. As I went over the nursing budget and staffing patterns, I was appalled by the unusually low number of graduate nurses and by the poor staffing during the evening and night shifts. I wanted to make a point of this in my report, so I tried to compare the actual number and type of nursing personnel budgeted and available with the minimum number that the associate director of nursing believed appropriate. It took me more than three days of review and discussion with this associate director before I could get her to outline for me (1) the many individual divisions of the hospital in which patients were cared for; (2) the approximate census that one might expect to budget or staff for; and (3) the minimal number of personnel who should be present for each shift. Whenever the director of nursing made up figures for each division and then extended it to the total number of nursing personnel that were required, we ran into a stone wall. She acknowledged that the figures were appropriate, but she would insist upon budgeting for far fewer personnel.

I finally understood the barrier regarding her formal budget request. The Cook County Board of Supervisors always refused to accept the number of personnel she thought proper because it would cost too much. Instead, they arbitrarily reduced the number of personnel. This had apparently happened so many times in the past that she had given up fighting for what she really believed was needed, and she just presented figures that she believed might be accepted. Ordinarily, my wife and I would have been critical of such an attitude, but it was clear that she knew what was needed and that she wasn't even aware of the mindset she had developed.

Another factor that impressed us as we haunted the emergency room evenings and weekends was the large number of patients that came there by ambulance via another hospital. Cook County Hospital had become a dumping ground for indigent patients in the Chicago area—even as many hospital leaders were advocating closing it down. Presbyterian-St. Luke's Hospital, virtually next door, was one of the strongest opponents of the continued existence of the hospital. And yet, as we sat in the ER, we saw patients being admitted who had come from the emergency room at Presbyterian-St. Luke's a few blocks away. Later, when we spent time visiting black areas of the city, my wife and I asked the residents why they did not go to their neighboring hospitals but went across town—sometimes via a complicated public transportation route—to get to Cook County Hospital. They often answered that they might have to wait, and the surroundings weren't attractive, but they would be getting the same care that everyone else was getting—whoever or whatever they were.

But the care at Cook County Hospital was not perfect. It was there that I was introduced to the so-called "All-American" operation, performed mainly on women for cancer and involving most of the organs in the abdomen and pelvis. I saw patients there with tubes in virtually every orifice, or with a leg disarticulated at the hip because of vascular complications (or mistakes) of surgery, lying helplessly in bed. Such matters did not lie specifically within my assignment, but I did not let the issue rest until I was satisfied that the hospital and its medical staff had established a professional and compassionate review mechanism to monitor all such procedures for the need as well as the competence of the physicians proposing to carry them out.

Mr. Ogilvie and I had a long discussion of the strengths and weaknesses of the institution. As expected, he asked me whether I would come to Chicago if he were able to carry out my recommendations, including that of taking control of the hospital away from the political Cook County Board of Supervisors and setting it up under a separate commission. I smilingly said no. I was then informed that I was to present my report formally to the Cook County Board of Supervisors in public session. This was an unexpected and unique experience. George Dunne, a powerful Democrat and the vice chairman of the commission, did most of the questioning. I told him what we saw as the strong and the weak points of the hospital, and I mentioned that one of the problems was political pressure on its staff and the expectation that they be loyal to and work for the political individual who had obtained them their jobs. Mr. Dunne skeptically questioned this. I responded that on election days, many of the hospital staff—particularly in the housekeeping, maintenance, and dietary departments—would not show up. Apparently they were required to work for their political sponsors on election day. If these individuals didn't carry out their political obligations, I said, their sponsor would withdraw his or her support and they would be "vised." Various members of the board indignantly denied the existence of such a procedure, and Mr. Dunne said he had never heard such a word. I replied that I had seen the payroll records of some employees who had been let go, and among the formal reasons for dismissal was sometimes written the word "vised." There were no more questions after that, and the meeting adjourned.

The following year, in my new position as coordinator of health services, I assisted with legislation that made the Cook County Hospital into a separate corporation. It was patterned after the Health and Hospitals Corporation in New York City and was theoretically free from political influence, but the board of supervisors still had financial control.

The only constant during the past fifteen years has been change. The governing board organization has been altered once more, and the institution is again the direct responsibility of the Cook County Board of Supervisors. Senior personnel management has changed, and there was a brief interlude in which the hospital had an operational contract with a hospital management firm. Its capacity has decreased, its physical plant has deteriorated. Current planning options vary from a complete replacement at the present site at a cost of $400–$500 million, to abandonment of the hospital.

A third alternative is the construction of a smaller unit in close proximity to the new University of Illinois Teaching Hospital. The unit would have approximately 450 beds and would share services and administration with the new hospital. Many of its special services are already handled by the University of Illinois Medical School faculty and resident staff, and $300 million in capital expense and perhaps as much as $25 million a year in operating expenses in the combined units could be saved, if appropriate services were combined. The problems of politics, patronage, job opportunities, unions, public relations, and professional support appear almost insurmountable—but perhaps the realities of limited financial resources will result in an innovative partnership of city, county, and state health resources.

THE COORDINATOR OF HEALTH SERVICES

I was flattered and pleased when Mr. Ogilvie, who had been elected governor of Illinois, asked me to be the coordinator of health services in the Office of the Governor. This was the first such position created by any governor in the United States. Wisconsin, Michigan, Pennsylvania and Kentucky tried it later with variations.

Early in his administration, Governor Ogilvie recognized the need for improved organization and administration in the state government. The number of agencies, departments, boards, commissions, committees and councils reporting directly to the chief executive made it difficult, if not impossible, for him to run an effective administration. As part of his 1969 executive reorganization, Governor Ogilvie created coordinator positions for several major areas of activity. The first of these was the coordinator of health services, established in August and filled by me in October of 1969. The coordinator was charged to counsel the governor on matters of health policy and to facilitate interagency health planning and administrative programs. Coordinators in manpower, conservation, and some social agencies were created later.

I had a small staff, but it was clearly understood that I was not responsible for any operations department and had no authority over any other agency. I frequently described my position as one with no authority but major authority. If I believed something should be done, I discussed it with the governor, and if he agreed it was appropriate he would follow through. I enjoyed myself in Illinois and gained cooperation from the directors and other individuals in the bureaucracy in part because I was meticulous about working with and through them. Only a few times in those four years did I ever directly approach the governor on any subject that had not already been explored in detail with the responsible directors.

The position of coordinator of health services is still difficult to define specifically. My understanding of the variety of approaches to health care did not really crystallize until I completed this experience, and, because the position was unique, I wanted to proceed slowly. During my term, I came to believe that health and social services were inextricably related, and I concluded that a state administration would be better served by a state division of health and social services or a state department for human services headed by a commissioner or director. As I look back upon the first year, I realize that I quickly started to consider eliminating my formal position in the state government. I saw the inherent danger of conflict between a staff individual and the various line officers, and I felt it would be appropriate to coordinate all of the health and social service activities under a single line executive, who could also assume my responsibilities as the governor's consultant. I took advantage of every opportunity to learn what other states were doing along these lines. I wanted to be able to recommend to the governor, when my four-year term was up, what I thought might be best for the future.

Mental Health

Shortly after I arrived in Chicago, I found my first semicrisis in the state health system. The director of mental health for the state had resigned to become chairman of the Department of Psychiatry in the Northwestern University School of Medicine. A search committee had been appointed to screen possibilities and make recommendations, and it had suggested two names. There was one rather major complication. Seven of the committee members favored one individual, and seven favored the other. However, there was one element of unanimity. All the committee members said that, if the governor selected the individual they opposed, they would vigorously fight against his programs.

I had met one of the committee members, who was dean of the Chicago Medical School and had been the chairman of its Department of Psychiatry when I had surveyed the Cook County Hospital. I asked him to help me with this dilemma. My first suggestion was that we thank the committee, dismiss all fourteen members, form a new committee, and appoint him chairman. In embarrassment, he explained to me that the fourteen committee members were the chairmen of the departments of psychiatry at the medical schools in Illinois—and one was the previous director of mental health. No other group of psychiatrists in Illinois could have the stature of this committee, and no psychiatrist of any standing or sense would want to serve in place of these eminent individuals. My next step was to invite the entire committee to my office. I laid forth the problem: they had come up with two individuals, each of whom half of them thought superlative and the other half despised. I knew neither candidate, but asked the committee members if they were being fair to them, the governor, or the mental health program in taking this rather arbitrary position. It was a fascinating meeting. Within an hour, they unanimously agreed that I should tell the governor that both candidates were appropriate and competent and that they would support whichever the governor selected. There was nothing magic in what I said or did. I was merely one professional bringing together a group of professionals and getting them to take a new look at the problem. The Governor finally selected Albert Glass from the University of Oklahoma as the new director.

I found, however, that the state mental health program had problems far more complicated than selecting a new director. Before my years in Illinois, and despite my previous experience with the Department of Mental Health in Connecticut, I was ignorant of the enormity, complexity, and importance of the mental health division in health and social services. In this I did not differ from most of my professional colleagues in medicine and health care administration. Not until I came to Illinois did I start to become aware of the role of mental health in the overall care of people, and of the breadth of its problems.

Before Dr. Glass got to Illinois, a major effort was being made to decrease the number and size of the state mental health hospitals and to stop "warehousing" mental patients. This all sounded reasonable to me, and I regret now that I paid relatively little attention to how it was being done. I knew of the advances in drug therapy for the mentally ill, but I was unaware that many of these patients could lead a more normal life in the community if properly followed on an outpatient basis. When I visited one of the state mental hospitals near Chicago, all I saw were the mechanics of discharge. The deputy director required that fifty to seventy-five patients a week be discharged into the community. The staff was having understandable difficulty with these quotas. However, I didn't discover until a year or so later that, while the discharging was done with relative efficiency, the arrangements for follow-up care were not properly made. All the discharged patients were housed in the Chicago community, but some enterprising entrepreneurs had bought up a number of apartment houses in north Chicago, and, in essence, were substituting apartment-house warehousing for institutional warehousing, with a minimum of psychiatric or social service follow-up. I was told that whole neighborhoods in north Chicago appeared to consist of these unfortunate ex-patients, either living in their apartment rooms or wandering forlornly on the streets.

States are now attempting to shift mental patients from large institutions to community-based centers, both ambulatory and in existing community hospitals, but the shift is still traumatic to the patients, the community, and the acute care hospitals. The State of Connecticut, for example, has closed whole institutions and has drastically reduced the capacity of others, presumably on grounds of economy and of providing more appropriate community facilities. But the acute care hospitals (many of which have added inpatient psychiatric services) are now finding that seriously ill or even disruptive or unmanageable psychiatric patients are brought to their emergency departments and must be kept in emergency rooms for several days because there is no room in the state psychiatric institutions. The hospitals are now appealing to the courts for assistance. Again the question arises: should mental health policy decisions in the state be made by health and social service professionals or by the budget office?

Cabinet for Health

A short time after I came to Illinois, the governor formally convened his Cabinet for Health, made up of the directors of Public Health, Mental Health, Public Welfare, Children and Family Services, the Bureau of the Budget, and a number of other state government divisions that had to do with health. The governor was chairman, and I served as secretary. John Dailey, one of the governor's administrative associates and the person with whom I worked most closely in the governor's office, was also part of this cabinet. My wife and I developed the agenda, which we then discussed with John Dailey. I tried hard to make sure that the topics on the agenda would be of interest or concern to most of the members, and I also tried to brief the governor before the meeting on the possible reactions and any differences of opinion likely to arise. In virtually every meeting at least one topic would lead to disagreements between two directors or one director or another would want to assume responsibility for a certain program or subject. I tried to anticipate these and have the topic introduced in such a way as to encourage open discussion and disagreement, if there were any. However, it was always clear that the final decision would not be made at the session. As a rule, the governor would hear the discussion, identify the disagreements, and then close the discussion by thanking individuals for their opinions and stating that he would decide later. He could thus decide for one department head and against another in private, so there would be no loss of face.

After the Cabinet for Health had been in place for about a year, the Governor called for a cabinet meeting on social services. The makeup of the two cabinets was essentially the same. From then on, we made no effort to differentiate—it was still called the Cabinet for Health, and its secretary was the coordinator for health services, but it demonstrated again the intimate relationship of health and social services in the state government.

The Nursing Home Scandal

Another example of the value of coordination of health and social service activities occurred during the *Chicago Tribune* expose of nursing homes in Illinois. My wife and I were in our Connecticut home for the weekend when I received a telephone call about the stories in the *Chicago Tribune*. The governor wanted me back for a special meeting of the Cabinet for Health the following day. We flew back to Chicago and I spent half the night on the telephone so that I could be at least somewhat informed at the meeting.

The Governor opened the meeting by expressing his concern over the stories which described poor food and care, overcharging, and abuse, and he asked what the truth of the situation was. He also asked for definition of the responsibilities of the various departments, how these responsibilities were being met, and what should be done about the allegations. The three departments involved were Public Health, which licensed nursing homes; Public Welfare, which paid for many nursing-home residents; and Mental Health, some of whose patients were in nursing homes. For the next hour, I was surprised and disappointed as the directors either ducked the issues or assured the governor that the accusations were exaggerated and that the nursing home situation was well in hand. From my own phone calls of the night before and from the comments of the directors, I knew that they were not familiar with the situation or were covering up. I passed a note to John Dailey, which said that they were trying to feed the governor a lot of baloney (I used a stronger expression). To my horror, Mr. Dailey passed my note to the governor, who read it without any change of expression. Shortly afterward, he adjourned the meeting, saying that he was still concerned about the *Tribune* reports and that I was to assume responsibility for following up. He instructed the directors of the three departments to cooperate.

I arranged for the senior deputy of each department to meet with me the following afternoon to pursue the matter in detail. I had met all three deputies and had been impressed with their dedication and knowledge of their departments. They had all been in the state service for years, so I was surprised when one of them thanked me for getting them together, saying this was the first time in his recollection that the three departments had been brought together formally to discuss mutual problems. It was a fascinating example of bureaucratic fragmentation.

The newspaper expose was published just prior to a meeting of the U.S. Senate Committee on Aging, which was coming to Chicago for hearings on nursing homes. I sat in on the hearings—the only one from the state government who sat there throughout the three-day period. Each of the directors testified, essentially repeating what they had told the governor, and, of course, I heard the representatives of the various nursing home groups defend themselves.

I wasn't sure whether the Office of the Governor should be publicly involved, so I just listened the first two days. Then I went to staff member Val Halamandaris and said I thought it would be appropriate for me to make some comments the next morning. I did so, stating that I believed many of the criticisms were justified, that the governor had discussed this with me and the directors, and that it would be explored in greater detail. I asked the Senate committee to come back at a later date, promising to present the details of our investigation and to report what we were doing to correct the deficiencies. The committee agreed. It was satisfying to see the various state departments affected and the nursing home directors and organizations work together constructively during the next few months. We were able at a subsequent hearing to state what we had found wrong and what we had done to correct the situation.

The CHP Advisory Board

The Governor and his aides originally told me that the staff of the state Comprehensive Health Planning Agency would be available to me for assistance. Some time after this, the agency director left, and the governor asked me to find a replacement. I discussed the job with a number of competent health planners whom I knew. I couldn't interest any of them in what they saw as a political position. The governor finally asked me to assume the responsibility. Long-time public health bureaucrat George Lindsley, who had been head of the Hill-Burton plan in Illinois and who had recently joined the Illinois Hospital Association was my executive officer—an unusually flexible and seasoned bureaucrat and an able staff associate. With his assistance we formed an advisory board representative of the state and of the various disciplines in health and social services. I confirmed the value of such professional and public input, particularly once the members realized that they were being asked to look at the problems of all the people in the state and not to function as special pleaders.

My experience with this representative board was quite different from that of many of my professional colleagues in planning agencies. Frequently they told me that their board members were nominated or appointed by a special group, and if they did not vote according to the party line they were replaced. I never had that problem and my procedure was relatively simple. I asked for recommendations from the various consumer and professional groups and made the appointments after making it as clear as possible to both the appointee and the group that appointed individuals brought the expertise or the experience of their groups but were themselves independent. Board meetings usually bore me to death, but I enjoyed these meetings—particularly when the public representatives reminded the health professionals that the people's needs were important.

The Illinois CHP Advisory Board provided me with a new educational experience. I had worked with various boards for years without giving any thought to whether board members participated at any personal sacrifice. After all, the board members with whom I usually dealt were professionals, executives, or spouses of prominent citizens. One of my prized CHP board members was Ellen Bohler, a nurses' aide in a state mental hospital and an eloquent advocate of the needs of people. When I called a board meeting, the organization paid the members' travel and living expenses, and most of the members continued to receive their salaries. But Ms. Bohler was not paid for the time she was absent from work. There were others like her, and my solution was simple: I approached each employer, explained that the employee was of value on a government assignment, and asked that the employer continue to pay his or her wages or salary. I obtained complete cooperation.

Bureaucracy and Politics

I had always considered *bureaucrat* a dirty word until I became one. The CHP staff, George Lindsley, and many other state employees were delightful surprises in their obvious desire to do a better job and help people. I particularly enjoyed George Lindsley's reaction whenever I came up with some new idea. He would tell me that it had never been done, and he didn't think it would be allowed. But he then went on to explore the idea, its rationale, and the objective, and then started working on the means by which the objective could be reached. I never felt that either yes-men or no-men were of much use, but I was pleased to find individuals who could tell me that something was against the rules or regulations or had never been done and then start trying to figure out how to accomplish it.

It took me months to appreciate my innocence in politics and bureaucracy. Shortly after I arrived in Illinois, I got into the habit of going down to the State Office Building on Saturday morning, dictating all my confidential memoranda on a Dictaphone belt, and then sending it air-mail to my secretary in Connecticut. I got it back typed and still confidential by Tuesday morning. The State Office Building on Saturday morning was like a mausoleum, unless the Governor was spending the weekend in Chicago. No offices were open, and there was only one elevator operator. I came to know all the elevator operators quite well. One day, one of them asked me if I were going to a certain barbecue. I didn't know anything about it. Then he asked me how much I had contributed to this event, and I said that I had given nothing. When we reached my floor, he kept on questioning me—he had made his contribution, and all his associates had, but I—one of the better-paid officials in the state—was apparently not making any political contribution. I said that I didn't believe in making such political contributions and if anybody asked me to do so I would tell him or her to go to hell.

About a year later I remarked to John Dailey that I had never been bothered with anyone concerned with political fundraising. He said, "You are unique. Before you came, the governor told us that you and your wife were coming here as professionals." The governor had apparently emphasized that we were not politically oriented in any way and had not been appointed for any political purpose. We were here to do a professional job in the field of health and were not to be approached under any circumstances for fundraising or political patronage. I confess that my opinion of Governor Ogilvie, already high, was raised even more.

Regionalization

I continued to learn about the leadership potentials in the governor's office and how simply and constructively it could be transmitted into action as the need arose. An early example was regionalization. Illinois, like virtually every other state, had many state departments whose subdivisions were usually developed to fit the needs of the particular department. Common regional boundaries existed only by happenstance. A constructive aspect of the CHP was the requirement that common state subdivisions be established for health planning.

As I became responsible for the development of the Regional Health Planning Agencies, I became aware of the variety of regional boundaries for the state agencies related to health. It seemed obviously advantageous to have uniform regions for all state agencies, not just those concerned with health. No one departmental commissioner, of course, had the authority to establish the jurisdiction or boundaries of any other department. But the Governor could exercise his authority through an executive order. I developed a rough outline of regional boundaries that appeared logical for the various departments, and I was able to get the directors and their deputies to compromise and adjust and finally to agree upon common boundaries, with certain exceptions here and there to meet brick-and-mortar realities. It was understood that regional boundaries were not immutable but that they could be changed only for logical reasons. I then presented our recommendations to the governor. The Cabinet for Health gave the plan a final review, and then the governor formalized the state's regions through an executive order. The whole process was accomplished rapidly and with a minimum of trauma.

The value of the common regions was demonstrated shortly before I left Illinois. One of the districts originally established was of twenty-seven counties in southern Illinois. The area was large, the population sparse, yet their problems with the state agencies were similar. Through the health planning agency I knew many of its departmental representatives for that region. They invited me to one of their offices to present a suggestion for consolidation, not of agencies, but of operations. The problem was that anyone in the region requiring services from different state agencies had to go to offices in two or three different towns, fill out separate forms asking for much of the same information but in different formats, encounter different criteria for acceptance or help, and, finally, put up with visits to his or her home by any of a number of agencies— frequently several in one day. These career bureaucrats complained of fragmentation, duplication, and inefficiency which they wanted eliminated. I applauded their analyses and urged them to fashion a simplified and efficient solution. One of my prized mementos from my four years in Illinois was their constructive report, which came from the state departments of Mental Health, Public Health, Public Aid, Children and Family Services, Vocational Rehabilitation, Corrections, the Governor's Office of Human Resources, the University of Illinois Extension Services and its Division for Crippled Children and Department of Community Development, and the Health Services Coordination Program of Southern Illinois.[8] I wish I could also say that their recommendations were implemented, but one of the hard realities of our political system is the lack of continuity in informed leadership and authority—particularly when the political party in power changes.

I found another challenging problem at the other end of Illinois, in Chicago, involving the provision of adequate health and social services to the more than one million blacks, Hispanics, and other minority groups in the city. I had no idea what was needed or how to help. Fortunately, my wife and I were able to recruit an associate, Catherine Stokes, a black Public Health nurse. She guided me in the vocabulary, economics, politics, and social health needs of a vitally important portion of Illinois's population. Another helpful associate was Obed Lopez, who persisted in developing a health clinic in Chicago despite frequent arrests by the Chicago police. I gather that his crime consisted of forming an independent neighborhood organization that might not be part of the established, politically approved system in Chicago.

Chicago Politics

Although I am sure that I seemed, to most individuals in Illinois, an innocent in politics, I wasn't totally blind to the political world around me. We knew of Mayor Daley and the Democrats in Chicago and that the governor of Illinois was a Republican. My relationships with Mayor Daley and his Health Department were almost entirely professional, but I shall never forget the day I went over to the office of the director of health, Murray Brown, and his deputy, Ed King, who functioned unofficially as the Mayor's representative in the department. I had a specific problem that I wanted to discuss, but shortly after I introduced it the deputy interrupted to congratulate me on my recently announced appointment as director of CHP. He went on to say that the CHP "b" Agency in Chicago, which was under my jurisdiction, could easily be taken over by the city Department of Health. This agency could be a valuable adjunct to the city and its Department of Health, he said, and if I helped arrange that, the city and Mayor Daley would be anxious to cooperate with me and the governor in many of the health activities throughout the rest of the state.

I stared at him in amazement, because this was the first time I had ever been approached about any type of political arrangement, and then

8. A. Snoke, "Health and Social Services in the State of Illinois: Report of the Ad Hoc Interagency Task Force of Southern Illinois to the Coordinator of Health Services." Report to the Governor, December, 1972, II, pp. 2–5.

started laughing. I said that I would no more suggest any type of political deal to the governor than I would fly, and that I had just finished Mike Royko's new book about Mayor Daley, *Boss*. There was still much amusement over the fact that Mrs. Daley had insisted that the book be taken off the shelf in a local store she frequented. When I finished my comments regarding politics and *Boss*, the deputy grinned and picked up the subject that I had originally come to talk about, and we went on from there.

Some time later, in the middle of the winter, as I was leaving our apartment building, the doorman asked if he could request a favor. He really didn't know what my position was in the state or the city, but he knew it had something to do with health and that I was tied in with the political world some way. Apparently the heating had broken down in his apartment house. The temperature was around zero, but the landlord appeared to be stalling. Was there anything I could do to help? I replied that I hadn't the slightest idea what could be done, but I would make some inquiries. When I got to the office, I called the city's deputy director of health and asked if I could come over and talk about a health problem in the city. Within ten minutes I was sitting in his office. I gave him the address of the building, the name of the landlord, and the situation as I understood it, and asked, "Is there anything from a health point of view that your department could do to check on this?"

The following morning the doorman stopped me and, with something like awe in his voice, reported on what had happened. By mid-afternoon, representatives from virtually every city department having to do with construction, sanitation, plumbing, wiring, and so on, had descended upon the apartment and interviewed the landlord. The landlord appeared duly impressed: the new boiler was being installed that day, and they expected to have heat by that night. I called the deputy director of health the next day to thank him, and reflected upon the power of government when it wanted something done, and the utter helplessness of the ordinary individual to influence such authority used, not used, or misused.

STATE ORGANIZATION FOR HUMAN SERVICES

My exposure to Chicago politics, and particularly my growing awareness of fragmentation and duplication of health and social services in the state, stimulated my search for a better human services system. I knew of the potentials and problems at the federal level, and I was of course familiar with the contributions of the private sector— particularly in health. Now I was learning firsthand that the state had certain responsibilities. But I wasn't sure what they were, and I also wasn't sure how the state should be organized to assume them. During our years in Illinois, my wife and I took every opportunity to visit other states to find out what they were doing, why, and how. Our first discovery was that most were like Illinois. They had the traditional departments of Public Health, Mental Health, Welfare, Children and Family Services, Crippled Children, Rehabilitation, Aging, and Correction, with few mechanisms for intercommunication. We saw this in Alaska, Oregon, California, Hawaii, Nebraska, and Connecticut. A second group of states had essentially the same organization and structure, but they were intrigued by Governor Ogilvie's creation of the position of coordinator of health services. I was asked to visit Wisconsin where Governor Patrick Lucey eventually created a similar position for a while. Governor William G. Milliken of Michigan sent a professor from Michigan State University to spend time with me exploring the idea for Michigan. Governor Milton J. Shapp of Pennsylvania asked me to come to Harrisburg, and he too subsequently created a position somewhat similar to mine.

Of all the states we visited, I was most impressed by Washington, and by the efforts of its governor, Daniel Evans, and the leadership of Charles Brink, dean of the School of Social Work at the University of Washington. Dean Brink, the governor's executive assistant, James Dolliver, and their associates were very frank in explaining to me their successes, problems, and failures. The fact that impressed me most, which was repeated in the experience of many states, was the time it took to plan, approve, enact, and implement a program. All emphasized that a complicated reorganization of state departments is not a one- or two-year development program but takes three to eight years. The continuation of the influence of any specific governor or administration obviously presents a problem, one that every state, as well as the federal government, must face, and the problem of continuity explains much of the futility of reorganization that we observed.

At this time I was introduced to the Council of State Governments in Lexington, Kentucky, and I learned of its reports on developing programs, organizational patterns, and administration in human services. I learned from the council as well as from individual states how jealously the various departments guarded their "turf," and how easy it was to thwart attempts at consolidation or cooperation by accusing its advocates of trying to form a "superagency," something apparently akin to the plague.

Massachusetts provided a beautiful example of the superagency for opponents of consolidation. There, advocates of greater coordination in health and social services had worked to create an efficient and stream-lined Office of Human Services. This new office was established within the state government by the legislature. Virtually every state agency, board, or commission that had anything to do with health or social services was declared to fall under the jurisdiction of the Executive Office of Human Services. These included departments of Public Health, Public Welfare, Mental Health, Correction, as well as numerous other boards and commissions dealing with youth, the aged, veterans, rehabilitation and rate setting. Having included all of these agencies, commissions, and departments in the new Executive Office of Human Services, the legis-lature then carefully added the restriction for each agency that "nothing in this section shall be construed as conferring any powers or imposing any duties upon the Secretary, with respect to the foregoing agencies, except as expressly provided by law." The legislature had listened carefully to the proponents of an improved organization for health and social services but even more carefully to the special interests, and it had, in fact, created a true superagency—which was not allowed to be organized into any effective or efficient human services department as originally desired. The Massachusetts superagency was described to me ad nauseam during my years in Illinois, for, despite the efforts of the governor of Mas-sachusetts and the recruitment of a number of able health administrators to press for legislation to organize the many independent agencies into an effective office, nothing much had been accomplished because of the necessity to protect departmental turf.

Connecticut provided another case history in the difficulty of state government reorganization. The Wilbur Cross Committee's efforts to reorganize the state government began in 1937, and the Chester Bowles Committee took on the challenge in 1950. I was not particularly impressed with the 1950 report, even when I reread it and found that listed as one of the senior consultants was one A. Snoke. While in Illinois, I had informal discussions with Connecticut governor Thomas Meskill's staff, and the inadequacies of the state's organization for people services was clearly recognized by both the Connecticut Etherington Commission Report of 1971 and the Zimmerman Commission Report to the Legislature in 1972. Both commissions recommended an integrated or consolidated admin-istrative structure for human services. The final result, substantially diluted by the legislature, was the Council on Human Services, created in the spring of 1973.

The original proposal suggested development of a single department of human resources, in which could be coordinated all the fragmented human services activities that presently existed in the state. But the final

Council of Human Services was effectively emasculated. Its first chairman frankly stated that no type of superagency would ever be advocated or allowed to result from the Council's activities. The Council on Human Services was allowed by the governor and the General Assembly to lapse into innocuous desuetude.

Connecticut tried again with the Filer Committee on the structure of state government, which presented its findings to Governor Ella T. Grasso in December, 1976. The report included specific recommendations on health and social services, but before it was even released publicly, Governor Grasso formally announced her opposition to any substantial reorganization of the departments related to human services—despite a devastating description of Connecticut's human services programs by Paul Nagle, for the Connecticut Association for Human Services, and the comments of the Filer Committee, which incorporated many of Mr. Nagle's findings in its formal report, and despite the fact that, during the previous seven to ten years, over twenty-six states had created relatively comprehensive human service agencies. Little progress in Connecticut can be reported since, other than Governor William O'Neill's January, 1985, statement that he intended to create a Cabinet-level position responsible for the twelve state agencies that administer human service programs. A coordinator of human services?

When I submitted my final report and recommendations to Governor Ogilvie at the end of 1972, I discovered that the governor's special advisor on state reorganization, John Briggs, after more than a year's study, had recommended the same type of human service reorganization as I had. Both of us favored a single state department for human services, with appropriate subdivisions, administered by health and welfare professionals but related closely to the larger department. But Mr. Ogilvie's term came to an end, and his successor, Democrat Daniel Walker, rejected any recommendations developed or sponsored by his predecessor. The coordinators of service positions were also abolished.

The reasons for lack of progress in state human service organization are many. One is the legitimate fear of the superagency that exists for the sake of its own being. Another is the selfish desire to protect turf, and a third the legitimate concerns of special interests which fear that whatever progress they have accomplished over the years will be lost in the broad picture. I sympathized with this concern at hearings where special groups, such as those representing the blind and the deaf, who had only recently obtained specific recognition in the state, voiced their fears of being again ignored. I can understand efforts to support an independent division for particular health or social services specialties in the state government and the protectiveness of those interested in such a division in the face of attempts to create an overall state administrative organization of human services. Individuals in each special category represent clearly the problems of ethics, philosophy, professional understanding, and leadership, the necessity of identifying the individual as a person, and the difficulties associated with limited economic resources. But preservation of the status quo will not solve the problems of fragmentation, duplication, waste, and inadequate care. Effective organization, administration, and leadership are required at all levels of government and in the private sector. The primary objective should be improving the health and welfare of *all* the people.

My experience over the years with the leadership of the PHS, HEW, and HHS, and particularly my involvement with state and regional administration, have led me to a number of convictions:

- Government is involved in the health and welfare of people, but the nature and extent of that involvement are still not clear—and will probably always be changing.
- The federal government cannot escape responsibility for developing a national human services policy and must play a major role in its financing.
- States must play a greater role in this collective responsibility for human services, because they are closer to the particular problems of their people. They, as well as the federal government, must improve organization, administration, leadership, and continuity—with fairness to the many unique sections of society that need and deserve consideration.
- The private sector involved with health and human services must be intimately involved with government as partners, rather than adversaries. This is an important and unique relationship, for in dealing with the health and welfare of the people the traditional goals of private enterprise, competition, and profit are not necessarily applicable.

These issues are currently being debated at every level from the individual provider to the federal administration. However, in the meantime, state governments should work more closely with the national organizations of governors, state governments, and state legislators. I can only offer my conviction that new leaders, legislators, and administrations should not automatically throw away everything that the previous party or individual did or believed in. For this reason I have advocated the formation of a nonpartisan, independent statewide Institution of Health that can bring together all of the forces related to health and welfare in a continuing cooperative organization.

I tried in 1976, under the auspices of the New Haven Foundation, and again in 1981, in association with the president of the Connecticut State Medical Society and the vice president for medical affairs of the University of Connecticut Medical Center, to form such an organization in Connecticut. Leaders of both medical centers (Yale and Connecticut), the Connecticut Medical and Hospital Associations, and state representatives from health and welfare, along with representatives from industry and insurance, met and as individuals expressed interest in and support for such an independent, widely representative organization. But reservations were expressed that such an organization might interfere with the dying CHP program, which was expected to be given a new lease on life by the new federal Health Systems Agency (HSA). At the second meeting, members were disillusioned about the possibilities of the HSAS, but no organization wanted to share in the expense of a new venture at the state level.

Today, the need for a prestigious, independent, authoritative, and objective organization broadly representative of all health and welfare components is great. The studies, evaluations, and recommendations it could generate would be of immeasurable value to the state. And certainly it would not be less productive than the continuing court battles of the hospitals and the Cost Control Commission, the perennial new state committees appointed to advise on reorganization, or the bland reliance on competition, marketing, strategic planning, and courts to solve all health care and social problems. We must get the many competing forces to face these complex issues as partners, not antagonists or competitors.[9]

9. A. Snoke and P. Snoke, "Linking Private, Public Energies in Health and Welfare Planning," *Hospitals* 16, 16 (August 16, 1976), 53–58.

10

Nursing

When I started out as an intern and a resident at Stanford, the prevailing doctrine held that nurses were the handmaidens of the doctors. I may have gone along, but I never quite accepted this stereotype. Even when I was a student I realized that the nurses educated me in people care as much as did my medical professors—if not more. And I always tried to work with nurses as partners and colleagues, not subordinates. One of the best nurses with whom I worked was the head nurse on the men's medical ward at Stanford University Hospital. A graduate of Stanford Nursing school, she was a full partner in patient care, obviously concerned with their welfare as well as the technical procedures ordered for them. She taught me how to do an abdominal paracentesis and also taught such procedures to my wife, who was interning the following year.

When I was on the resident staff in pediatrics at Stanford, the head nurse and the social worker were my primary instructors in the practical and personal problems of children and their parents. I collaborated in the same way with the pediatric nurses and social workers during my final residency year in Rochester. At Stanford, the value of the personal influence of nurses upon patients, as contrasted to a scientific, intellectual approach, was impressed on me in one series of episodes. A socially prominent San Franciscan periodically showed up or was brought roaring drunk to the psychiatric unit. No one could approach him with any type of tranquilizer but Margaret (Maggie) Rouse, the head of the division. Although Maggie was under five feet tall and he was over six feet, she had his confidence and respect. He meekly obeyed her, took the paraldehyde that was routinely given at that time, and behaved as she told him until discharge.

The idea of the nurse as a handmaiden of the physician was deeply rooted in the medical profession. At first, I accepted without question that the nurse at the desk would stand up when a physician approached her— no matter what she was doing—but this practice soon made me uncomfortable. We eliminated it before I left Rochester, and when I came to New Haven I found it had been abolished for years—probably due to the influence of Annie Goodrich and Effie Taylor.

As I became acquainted with a number of distinguished hospital administrators, I realized that administrative ability was not a sex-linked characteristic. One such episode is clearly etched in my memory. A few weeks after I came to New Haven, Francis Blake, the dean of the medical school and chairman of the Department of Medicine, told me that he had heard a number of complaints about the director of nurses, Laura Grant, and he suggested that I consider discharging her. As he detailed the criticisms, I noticed that they sounded similar to those I used to hear from the faculty in Rochester about the director of nurses there, Clare Dennison. I told him that I had worked closely with her, admired her, and had been skeptical of my academic colleagues' evaluations. However, inasmuch as I was new in New Haven, I would proceed slowly and consider his advice seriously.

Shortly after this conversation, I visited Miss Grant's office. I saw the *Wall Street Journal* on her desk. I didn't know anyone who subscribed to the *Journal*, and I expressed interest and surprise. Oh yes, she read it regularly. Later we got into a discussion involving calculations, and as I started to multiply and divide laboriously she pulled out a slide rule and promptly came up with the answer. I had tried since college to learn the "slip-stick" but never had. Afterward, I returned to my office and laughed at myself. Laura Grant was one of those superb women, like Clare Dennison, Anne Ryle, Kate Hyder, Ruth Sleeper, Lucille Petrie Leone, Annie Goodrich, and Elizabeth Bixler, who taught me the value of the nurse in patient care. No handmaidens these.

I did not pay much attention to the economic exploitation of nurses and the condescending attitudes of many physicians until I had spent some ten years in hospital administration. I never realized during this period that we were exploiting the student nurses, although frequently their workday started at seven in the morning and ended at seven or eight at night, with time off during the middle of the day. I had followed a similar schedule during my five years of internship and residency—except that I didn't have any time off—and it was what most nursing educators and hospital administrators were accustomed to, so it raised no eyebrows.

In New Haven, the Yale School of Nursing graduate program sharply distinguished between clinical supervisors and nursing teaching supervisors, the latter of which had not existed in Rochester or Stanford. The hospital was responsible for service; the nursing school for teaching. When the Grace-New Haven School of Nursing diploma program moved into the new hospital in 1953, the same separation of supervisors prevailed. As a result, the hours of service required of nursing students were reduced. I disapproved at first, but after observing the instruction and realizing the need for the students to be properly educated, I was convinced that the nursing educators were correct. However, at Yale we continued to exploit student nurses, graduate nurses, and other hospital employees—particularly women—for many years. Correcting this has played a major and sometimes unadmitted role in increasing hospital costs, and it should be taken into account in analyses of these cost increases over the past twenty-five years.

I am still pleased that I was smart enough in 1951 to establish Anne Ryle as a director, and formally a part of the hospital administration, instead of just the department head for nursing. Even though the head of nursing has the toughest job in the hospital, it took hospitals years to regard, as well as to reward, these individuals properly. Miss Ryle had to administer the largest single operational unit in the hospital. Although she was responsible to the hospital administrator, her nursing personnel had to report not only to her, but also to the resident staff and the attending physician. The latter usually felt they were responsible to no one. However, although I recognize the value of administration in nursing, it took me longer to accept the idea that becoming an administrator might not be the only legitimate way for a nurse to earn more money. At first, a nurse could only increase his or her salary by becoming assistant head nurse, head nurse, supervisor, or administrator. Only years later did we begin to understand that better bedside nurses, nurse midwives, and nurse practitioners also deserved better pay. Now administrators are working on differentiating between levels of training, experience, and responsibility and granting status and salary accordingly.

Those in the nursing program who correlate administrative ability and competence with a ph.d. degree are making a similar mistake. One prestigious medical center kept a highly regarded nurse in an acting chief capacity for three or four years only because she did not possess a ph.d. I can only repeat what I have said about an m.d. degree: since when does either an m.d. or a ph.d. guarantee administrative ability or common sense?

NURSING EDUCATION AND RESPONSIBILITY

I never really understood nursing education, but this never used to bother me. It was not my responsibility, and there were a lot of other things I didn't understand. However, as a hospital administrator, and later as I got involved in health care administration outside the institution, I became more aware of the various types of professional skills needed to care for people. And as I became more closely associated with the leaders in the American Nursing Association (ANA) and the National League for Nursing (NLN), as well as the directors of the nursing programs related to my own medical center, I got the uncomfortable feeling that many nursing leaders still did not agree about what nursing education should be or about what nurses could or should do.

Grace-New Haven was the host to educational programs for nurses' aides, licensed practical nurses, hospital diploma nurses, and baccalaureate nurses. It also provided the clinical facility for the Yale University School of Nursing, which for years had admitted students who already had a baccalaureate degree. After a twenty-four to twenty-eight month educational period, they were awarded, through 1936, a Bachelor of Nursing degree and, through 1958, a Master of Nursing. There were authoritative and respected advocates among my associates for each program and each level of nursing. I learned later of the proposed two-tier associate degree program in a junior college, which was introduced to me by Mildred Montag of the Teacher's College at Columbia, in 1952. The difference in opinion regarding nursing service and education do not seem to have been settled. I suspect that many nursing leaders are acting just like my physician colleagues, looking at their roles and responsibilities in relation to what they consider to be the best interests of their profession. I cannot fault them—I do the same. But these groups must also consider the need to provide for total patient care.

This concept brings in the philosophy of levels of care. All patients are not acutely ill, and the philosophy of a continuum of care acknowledges that many individuals, both within and outside of the hospital, can be cared for by less highly trained personnel. For years, I could not have operated Grace-New Haven without these lower-paid nursing personnel. But the role of the nurse and his or her associates changed over the years, as did our patients' needs, and, by the time I left the hospital in 1968, almost half the patients on our service divisions could be classified for intensive care and needed the kind of nursing that only highly skilled personnel could provide. The less highly trained nurses no longer met their needs.

As the role of the nurse, and overall medical and social needs has changed, I have wondered whether the educational philosophy in the health professions reflects the need for people care or overemphasizes the acute care environment. The challenge facing nursing leaders is the same as that facing medical educators. Are they organizing the educational environment to provide students experience with the continuum of care, or are they overemphasizing the more exciting acute phases of illness? There are many cogent arguments for the continuum of care philosophy: rising health costs will force us to use less expensive personnel when possible and to train individuals with varying levels of skill for the different types of care; professionals must learn to employ a team approach to obtain optimum results across the spectrum of care. It is more efficient to provide services in a team approach rather than through separate, fragmented service entities. This has long been my own goal in health care, and it is even more vitally necessary today, although it is more difficult now than yesterday and will be even more difficult tomorrow.

Most patients have little understanding of the various levels of nursing education. As a patient, I was always delighted when nurses came around, but I frequently hadn't the slightest idea whether the nurse had a master's or a baccalaureate, or whether he or she was a diploma school graduate or an LPN. Of course I wanted the correct medication and wanted my condition monitored professionally. But I also wanted to be comfortable. In my hospital experiences, the most satisfying care I had was given by a strong, gentle LPN who could make me comfortable and taught my wife to help me move in bed. Of course highly educated nurses are needed to listen to and interpret patients' needs and concerns to the attending physician or the resident staff. But the personality and interest of the nursing personnel in the individual patient are just as important as training, if not more so. Experience, knowledge, understanding, and sympathy directed to their patients' fears, worries, and personal needs are far more important to sick people than the names of the degrees on the nurse's curriculum vitae. I suspect the public is more aware of this unique human contribution of the nurse than many of us realize.

THE YALE UNIVERSITY SCHOOL OF NURSING

I have never encountered a more perceptive and competent group of nurses than those who received the degree of Master in Nursing from the Yale University School of Nursing from the 1930s to the 1950s. But Yale's president abolished the program in 1956, because in his view it was not a true master's program but merely a training program for selected individuals who had already received a baccalaureate degree in some other subject. I argued heatedly with him when he told me, only two days before the announcement, about his intention—but I only had examples and descriptions of the graduates' superb capacity, whereas he had the authority of his position, backed up by the opinions of two consultants. One was the president of a prestigious women's college in the East. The other was the dean of an equally prestigious medical school. That neither individual had any knowledge of nursing responsibilities or education meant little to President Griswold. They were respected members of academe. I was particularly surprised by the action because the president's executive assistant had been chairing a special committee on the academic reorganization of the nursing school for the past year. Years later I learned that members of the faculty of the Yale Medical School—including its dean—had been critical of the nursing school.[1] I also learned many years later that this attitude had existed in Rochester around 1950, when some faculty members of the school of medicine expressed violent opposition toward granting academic recognition to the faculty of the School of Nursing at Strong Memorial Hospital.[2] It has taken a long time to convince some doctors that nurses are also professionals!

Fortunately, vestiges of the Yale nursing program remained, and an academic master's program was established in 1960.

NURSES, PHYSICIANS, AND THE CONTINUUM OF CARE

The role of the nurse as an individual, independent practitioner had not truly developed—was not even much considered, with the possible exception of midwifery—by the time I left hospital administration. But as an administrator I was impressed with the nurse midwives, and I came to appreciate greatly the roles of the public health nurse, visiting nurse, or home health care nurse during my work with the Regional Visiting Nurse Agency (RVNA). I was impressed with their practical knowledge of the handling of patients in the home, their responsibility for considering that patient's overall needs, and their recognition of the necessity to involve other professional disciplines. And I was often surprised at how little the attending physician really knew of the personal problems of his or her patients, problems that in many cases overshadowed their purely medical ones. However, as I watched these nurses work with patients, involving social workers, dieticians, the physical therapists, and other specialized personnel in their care, I became convinced of the need for an overall director or coordinator. Ideally this should be the physician—but most physicians still don't have a true understanding of the problems faced by

1. Dorothy A. Sheehan, "A Social Origin of American Nursing and Its Movement into the University: A Microscopic Approach," Ph.D. diss., New York University School of Education, 1980.
2. The University of Rochester Medical Center: To Each His Farthest Star, 1975, 199.

patients outside the hospital. As pressures mount to discharge patients from the acute care hospital earlier, home health care personnel will be faced with the need to perform more complicated procedures. The education of these caretakers must be superb and their relationships with the physician close. The opposite is also true: the physician must become aware of the potential of home care and the whole patient environment. A mutual education program is thus necessary, in which the physician must learn how to delegate responsibility and depend upon the skilled nurse in the home, while the nurse improves and expands his or her skills in order to assume this responsibility and work closely with the physician. This will require education and training, experience and perceptiveness, and obviously the best academic training possible. Whether the physician becomes a narrower specialist or assumes a broader responsibility for overall patient care, the nurse will prove of even greater value if he or she brings a perceptive concern for overall patient care to the team. Thus I come back to my comment that nursing educators need to be reminded of the continuum of health and care. As we come to understand better the gradations of health, we can tailor the gradations in the education required for nursing personnel. This is important from a financial as well as a professional point of view. Learning how and when to rely on less highly trained personnel should be a fundamental part of the education of physicians and nurses. For example, in many cases, a skilled professional will be needed with special education in geriatrics as well as psychiatric nursing. In others, an LPN, home health aide, or homemaker will be all that is required. Professional educators must realize the differing service needs and organize their educational and service programs accordingly.

11

Aging, Medicare, and Home Health Care

The history of care for the aged is as descriptive of the transition in the care of people in our society as any other example with which I am familiar. Medical attitudes in the 1930s were personally sympathetic and professionally fatalistic. The treatment of an elderly person with acute heart disease, malignancy, or acute degenerative disease was seen as a challenge, but we had no solutions for long-term, chronic problems, beyond waiting for the inevitable end. Unfortunately, caring for a patient with a chronic, progressive disease was not very exciting. These were the "crocks"—a term that should have disappeared long ago from the health vocabulary, but it persists. We still move slowly in our understanding of the needs of the chronically ill and aged. Allen Spiegel, in his excellent 1983 book on home health care,[1] quotes *Les Misérables* to illustrate society's and physicians' disinterest in the care of the aged: "The misery of a child is interesting to a mother; the misery of a young man is interesting to a young woman; the misery of an old man is interesting to nobody."

As a medical student or house officer, I had little knowledge or interest in the nonmedical problems of the elderly—and there was little in my first years of hospital administration that prompted me to pay much more attention to them. The delivery of health care to the acutely ill was a personal challenge to me and my associates, but long-term care, custodial facilities, and their financing were someone else's concern. During the 1950s, I slowly became aware of chronic disease and aging when, as

1. A. D. Spiegel, *Home Healthcare: Home Birthing to Hospice Care*. Owings Mill, Md.: National Health Publishing, 1983.

184

executive director of Grace-New Haven, I received several requests a week for the name of a physician to take care of some patient. I usually tried to match the patient with the physician I considered most appropriate. There were two internists in New Haven, Howard Colwell and Allen Poole, for whom I had great respect as thoughtful, sympathetic physicians, and I almost inevitably referred the older patients to one of these two, because of their rapport with and support of the elderly.

Meanwhile, health care for the elderly was becoming a major political and health issue—primarily focused on the financing of that care. The several Wagner-Murray-Dingell bills, legislation supported by Representative Aime Forand of Rhode Island, the King-Anderson bill, and the Kerr-Mills bill were all evidence of a growing national interest in aging. The elderly, however, continued to have difficulty finding health professionals to deal with their problems, and they were still unable to generate sufficient power and authority to have their specific needs understood and met. My wife's and my follow-up study of the Kerr-Mills bill for the aged[2] and my continuing confrontation with organized medicine and the hospital-based specialties in the years prior to the passage of Medicare in 1965 first pushed me toward concern with health care for the aged. To be honest, however, I was primarily involved with the financial, administrative, and political aspects of that health care. The professional challenge and responsibility involved in care of the aged was still not of special interest to me.

Following the legislative battles that belatedly made me conscious of the health problems of the aged, my wife and I visited England in 1967 and 1969, where we combined sightseeing with a study of the British health system. One of our most intriguing discoveries was that, of the various medical specialties formally functioning in the British system, geriatricians numbered only a few less than pediatricians. I didn't know one doctor in Rochester or New Haven who was classified as a geriatrician.

One experience in Illinois was even more enlightening. Shortly after we arrived in 1969, we learned that the only relative of a close friend of ours from overseas had been in a mental institution in Illinois for some time, with a diagnosis of "senility." We visited her and discovered that she—like the other 39 women in that division—was bedridden and could not move. The doctors and nurses frankly told us that most of their patients were merely old, with varying degrees of "senility." The patients had all been ambulatory when they arrived, but after being put in bed

2. A. Snoke and P. Snoke, "Health Care of the Aged," *Connecticut Medicine* 27, 11 (1963), 679–83; A. Snoke and P. Snoke, "How Kerr-Mills Works in Connecticut," *The Modern Hospital* 101, 2 (August, 1963), 79–82, 154–57.

they had lost their mobility and now were completely bedridden. They also described a change in treatment over the past year. Similar patients were being kept ambulatory in a separate unit, and the staff was proud of the fact that few of the new patients were bedridden. This experience came at just the right time to help me solve another problem that was facing Illinois and other states: the decreasing need for hospitalization for tuberculosis, and the decreasing census of the Illinois State Tuberculosis Hospital in Chicago. My wife and I commuted from Chicago to Springfield once or twice a week, and, one morning, Dr. Glass, the director of mental health for Illinois, was on the plane with us. I needled him about the large number of elderly people that were being admitted to state mental institutions—why did staff accept patients who were not really psychiatric cases but just old or making trouble for their families? Dr. Glass agreed completely with my criticism both of the inappropriate use of mental institutions and of the stigmatization endured by these patients who were not mentally ill. But what in blazes could he do about it when the patients appeared as the result of family requests and physician referrals? I suddenly had the idea of using part of the tuberculosis hospital as a screening institution for this type of patient.

Unfortunately, the noise level in this commuter plane was high, and both Dr. Glass and I had to yell to make our voices heard. (Neither of us was a particularly quiet individual anyway.) My wife kept trying to quiet us down because the other passengers seemed fascinated by this noisy discussion. But we paid no attention to her admonition, and by the time we had landed in Springfield we had a proposal for the Governor. We suggested converting sixty beds in the tuberculosis sanitorium into a diagnostic unit for all elderly patients referred to northern Illinois state mental institutions, unless they were clearly psychotic. We would staff the screening unit with the faculty of the nearby University of Illinois Medical School, and make the unit the responsibility of the Illinois Department of Public Health, rather than the Department of Mental Health, so as to remove any possible stigma.

The new unit was in operation within a few months. Its first year proved rather startling. A few of the patients were found to have malignancies or other terminal diseases for which nothing could be done but palliation. A considerable number were found to have nutritional or other remedial conditions and could be treated and returned home. Others were admitted to nursing or convalescent homes. Fewer than 10 percent of those admitted to the screening unit were eventually committed to mental institutions. The program and the unit were discontinued some years later for reasons that were not entirely clear, but probably a combination of shifting organization and responsibility as well as the changing interest of those responsible. Academic or professional interest in geriatrics did not really appear in Illinois until the early 1980s. The University of Illinois Health Sciences Center has only recently expanded its program and leadership in this field. Some type of a geriatric unit will undoubtedly emerge in that complex.

My early experience with the evaluation for the aged, plus the *Chicago Tribune* exposé of nursing homes and the hearing held by the Senate Committee on the Aged (discussed in chapter 9) prompted me to follow through on the state's activity on this subject. I found that the official state division concerned with the aged consisted of four rather elderly persons, one of whom was Elizabeth Breckenridge. I started to learn from her about the social and health problems of the aged, but unfortunately, and despite their complexity, their problems were of minor importance in the state at that time.

My wife and I left Illinois in 1973 with the uncomfortable feeling that the major social and health problems of the aged were being inadequately addressed, despite the voices purporting to speak for the elderly in Washington and in various special interest groups. Our feeling was not diminished when, at the Association of American Medical Colleges (AAMC) meeting in 1978, we heard Paul Beeson deliver the first report of his special committee organized by the Institute of Medicine in response to a request from the director of the National Institute on Aging that a study be made of incorporating aging into American medical education.[3] Dr. Beeson's presentation was authoritative and sobering. He pointed out that at the turn of the century, only 4 percent of Americans were older than sixty-five. In 1978, the figure was about 11 percent, and by the end of the century it is expected to be much higher. The U.S. Bureau of the Census estimates that, by the year 2020, 17.3 percent of the population will be over sixty-five years of age. It also estimates that the actual numbers of those over sixty-five will increase, from 25 million in 1980 to 51 million in 2020.[4] Recognizing that the aged require much health care, Dr. Beeson estimated that approximately 50 percent of this nation's health costs and 50 percent of physicians' time will be devoted to this relatively small proportion of the total population. Even with these projections, Dr. Beeson declined at that time to advocate any specific specialty such as geriatrics or gerontology, but rather urged that the responsibility be

3. Paul Beeson, AAMC-CA Talk on Aging, AAMC annual meeting, New Orleans, October 28, 1978.

4. U.S. Bureau of the Census, "Aging America—Trends and Projections," ser. P-25, no. 922, October, 1982.

assumed by internists, general practitioners, or family physicians. However, he did remind the medical educators at the meeting that students now in their classes and on their resident staffs would be responsible for caring for these people in the year 2000. What were they doing now to prepare these doctors of the future for this responsibility? A series of articles in the June, 1981 issue of the AAMC *Journal of Medical Education* gave a preliminary report on how this challenge had been responded to.[5] The results were not encouraging. More interest was being shown by 1985, but it is still a gradual process.

I was exposed further to health care for the aged when I became involved with the Regional Visiting Nurse Agency (RVNA), a home health care agency for four towns on the periphery of New Haven. In 1984, 69 percent of its case load were patients over sixty-five years of age, and 49 percent were over seventy-five. In Hamden, the largest of the four towns they served, more than 23 percent of the population was over sixty. Because I was suspicious of the health and social programs for the aged in the region and the state—suspecting duplication and fragmentation as well as deficiencies in service—I encouraged Claudia Smith, a student in Yale's Department of Epidemiology and Public Health, to devote her master's thesis to the subject of care for the aged in the region. The thesis, completed in the fall of 1983, did little to relieve my concern.[6] Nor were the additional facts on Medicare and the health costs of the elderly presented to the Senate's Special Committee on Aging in April, 1984, encouraging.[7] The report to the Special Committee emphasized the high percentage of Medicare funds used by a relatively low percentage of the elderly—those in the last six-to-twelve months of life and particularly those in the terminal stages. The report also described the high percentage of Medicare reimbursement for hospital care (almost two-thirds), the high percentage of the cost of illness or disability that was still being borne by the elderly, and the inadequacies of Medicaid in helping the elderly poor. Claudia Smith's thesis also documented the variety of services needed by the elderly. She found a "crazy quilt of services available to the elderly" in the four towns studied, which illustrated how dependent health and social services were upon the amount, type, and condition of available funds. As I tried to match the needs of the elderly with the services and funds available, I was reminded how dollars and disease had been my own priorities until I finally recognized the social needs, as well

5. "Geriatrics and Medical Education," *Journal of Medical Education* 56, 6 (June, 1981).

6. C. Smith, "Services for the Elderly," Master's Thesis, Yale University, 1983.

7. Senate Special Committee on Aging, "Medicare and the Health Costs of Older Americans: the Extent and Effect of Cost Sharing," April 1984.

as the health needs, of the aged. I also realized how slow my professional colleagues and I had been in getting the program started, and how money always seemed to be the top priority.

MEDICARE

Medicare was, of course, a major step taken toward the goal of meeting the health care needs of the aged. My participation in the development and implementation of the national Medicare legislation in 1965 was a logical extension of my activities in health care and hospital administration up to that time. I had never before been personally involved in national health legislation. Even when I was in the top of the AHA hierarchy in the late 1950s, Edwin Crosby and his staff—particularly Kenneth Williamson—handled the hospitals' interests in Washington.

By the early 1960s, medical care for the aged had become a major issue, both politically and in the private sector. Specific legislation, leading to the Medicare Act in 1965, brought into sharp focus the philosophical and organizational differences between, on the one hand, organized medicine (the AMA) and the organized hospital-based specialists, and, on the other, the AHA, the state hospital associations, and the hospital administrators. Although these differences had existed for at least twenty-five years, they had usually been of relatively short duration. The AMA and AHA leaders and their senior staff were usually able to discuss and compromise. Unfortunately, the issues that were presumably resolved in this manner seemed always to be challenged later by a dissenting special interest. Federal health programs were always regarded with suspicion by organized medicine—and to a lesser extent by hospitals—but as long as they were confined to selected areas, such as financing for hospital construction, the Servicemen's Dependents' Health Program, care of children and mothers during the war (EMIC), or the Veterans' Administration, no substantial objections were raised. Any national health program for the populace as a whole, however, was fiercely resisted. This was evinced by the AMA's reaction in 1932 to the report of Ray Lyman Wilbur's Committee on the Cost of Medical Care, the series of Wagner-Murray-Dingell bills starting in 1943, and the efforts of presidents Roosevelt, Truman, Eisenhower, Kennedy, and Johnson to develop national health legislation.

The AMA's 1932 reaction is worth recalling. In an editorial, Morris Fishbein wrote that the issue was clear: "On the one side, the forces representing the great foundations, public health officialdom, social theory—even socialism and communism—inciting to revolution; on the other side, the organized medical profession of this country, urging an orderly evolution, guided by controlled experimentations, which will observe the principles that have been found through the centuries to be necessary to the sound practice of medicine."[8] By 1960 the problems of health care for the aging population were becoming a matter of great concern, not only to older people themselves, their families, and the population in general, but also to health administrators, Blue Cross and commercial insurance programs, health and welfare organizations, and medical and social politicians. The whole subject was so complex that the issues became oversimplified to a choice between complete medical and hospital care financed by the federal government ("socialized medicine!") or the preservation of private practice, voluntary hospitals, rugged individualism, and private enterprise. The federal program became categorized as "the King-Anderson approach," and the private program was called "the Kerr-Mills approach." The American Nursing Association and the American Public Health Association publicly espoused the former, the American Medical Association and the AHA the latter.

My wife and I studied the Kerr-Mills program in Connecticut. As might be expected, we found that its solemnly uttered principles and beliefs differed markedly from reality. While the national bill presented basic standards, every state had variations in its local implementing legislation. Eligibility, benefits, and caseloads varied from state to state. And relationships to other state health and welfare programs were so complicated that it was very difficult to reach any firm conclusion about how this national policy was affecting the states. Nevertheless, we learned several things. Alert state administrations could shift *their* existing financial obligations to care for patients under Old Age Assistance (OAA) to the federal government by transferring OAA patients to Kerr-Mills. This was done very successfully in Massachusetts, New York, Connecticut, and in a few other states, so that federal financing became a major factor in the health care of the aged in those states. We never figured out why more states did not take advantage of this opportunity to shift state expenditures to the federal level.

We also learned that, in states with large Kerr-Mills programs, virtually everyone concerned (including physicians) pushed for less strict eligibility limits and for elimination of the hundred-dollar deductible. There was also pressure to get Kerr-Mills to pay professional fees for medical services rendered by private physicians. This was written into the Connecticut law at the request of the Connecticut State Medical Society. Their professional fees came from federal funds—presumably cleansed of

8. M. Fishbein, *jama* 99, 23 (1932): 1950–52.

any association with socialized medicine by passing through state channels. For some reason, organized medicine never officially recognized the important role of the federal government in Kerr-Mills financing.

While these events were occurring at the local and state levels, activity was increasing at the national level. During 1961, I participated in a series of joint meetings of representatives of the AMA and AHA boards, held to explore the possibility of developing a joint statement of principles. After considerable discussion that led nowhere, Kenneth Williamson, head of the AHA's Washington office, and I retired to try to write a statement that the two bodies might agree upon. The basic principles were that health care for the aged was expensive, that they did not have the financial resources to pay for it themselves, that the private sector could not underwrite the expense either, and that some sort of financial assistance from government was thus necessary and indicated. But the AMA representatives would not accept any statement that implied that government—particularly federal—funds were necessary or acceptable, nor were they certain they could accept the fact that the elderly needed financial help. This marked the beginning of a very sharp break in attitude and organizational posture between the two organizations. Beginning with Williamson's and my preliminary statement, the AHA developed a formal statement of policy, which was presented to its House of Delegates and the member plans of the Blue Cross Association in a special combined meeting in January, 1962.[9]

This policy statement was not very different from that developed by Williamson and me but it did state specifically that the source of the government assistance was of secondary importance to the AHA. The special meeting on the subject in 1962 was one of the most extraordinary I have ever attended. I sat near Alanson Willcox, who had been general counsel for the AHA and was now the general counsel for HEW, and Joseph Stetler, then general counsel for the AMA and later the president of the American Pharmaceutical Association. Both of them could scarcely contain themselves during the considerable debate by the AHA delegates. A number of the states, notably West Virginia and New York, expressed considerable dissatisfaction with the Kerr-Mills program—many states were not even participating. No one, however, disagreed with the fact that the elderly needed assistance in financing their health care.

The most fascinating part of the session, however, was the appearance of F. J. L. (Bing) Blasingame, the executive vice president of the AMA, who spoke to the House of Delegates during the luncheon

9. Special Meeting of the American Hospital Association's House of Delegates and the Member Plans Blue Cross Association, Chicago, January 3–4, 1962, AHA Minutes.

recess. Dr. Blasingame did not confine his remarks to an expression of the
AMA's opposition to federal participation in financing health care for the
aged, but went on to denounce the proposed recommendations and even
threatened reprisal by local physicians and hospital boards against individual administrators if the recommendations were passed. I was very
proud of the House of Delegates' reaction. They knew that Dr. Blasingame
had made no idle threat, and there was no question that many hospital
administrators were vulnerable to criticism from the organized medical
staff. Nevertheless, the House of Delegates endorsed by a very substantial margin the recommendations. Federal participation in financing
health care for the aged was a key factor in what eventually appeared in
1965 as Title XVIII or Medicare.

I had nothing to do with the preparation of the Medicare legislation,
but I still recall watching on television the massive Madison Square
Garden assembly of May 20, 1962, with thousands waving banners and
applauding speeches favoring the development of a national health program for the elderly—and the broadcast on the following night in which
Edward R. Annis (president of the AMA in 1963–64) spoke. With the
ribbons, papers, and signs from the previous night's rally still cluttering
the seats and the floor, Dr. Annis denied the need for any type of federal
health program for the aged. (He did, however, strongly advocate the
Kerr-Mills approach, which many had found unsatisfactory—and he
ignored the role of the federal government in its financing.)

Although skirmishing continued between the AMA and AHA, the
primary activity was now in Washington, D.C. It became increasingly
clear that there was momentum toward national legislation to provide
hospital costs for the aged. The next development was the proposal that
national health insurance pay for hospital care (part A of the eventual
Medicare legislation) and also partially pay for medical costs (part B of
Medicare). This concept was embraced by Wilbur Mills, chairman of the
House Committee on Ways and Means. The result was mandatory hospital insurance for the elderly and the semblance of a voluntary, contrib-
utory medical insurance program under government auspices. Part B
required a patient's willingness to have part of the cost deducted from his
or her Social Security payment. There would also be an annual deductible
and a co-insurance factor which would require the patient to pay 20
percent of the professional fee paid by Medicare. The government would
pay for the hospital costs (part A) from Social Security payroll tax revenue. I was surprised to hear of the addition of the medical component to
the national health insurance program, and I gather that the AMA was also.
But, so long as it resulted in an acceptable national health insurance
program for the aged, it was fine with me—except that the part B provi-

sions were rather complicated and difficult to understand. The proposals appeared to accommodate the variety of existing hospital-specialist arrangements of billing and reimbursement.

Some time later, I received an emergency telephone call. It was from Kenneth Williamson of the AHA, telling me that Mills had had the Medicare bill altered so that all of the hospital-based specialty services were covered under part B of the proposed law—the one requiring deductibles and co-insurance. I felt as if I had been transported back twenty years in my administrative relationships with organized medicine, the specialists, and the principles of third-party reimbursement. I was not privy to the development in Washington that had caused the shift of hospital-based specialties from hospital-based reimbursement to medical-based reimbursement. I learned later how representatives of the hospital-based specialties had worked with the AMA to make the change. Their position was that, if a national health insurance for the aged was inevitable and there was to be provision for the payment of physicians, all physicians should be reimbursed in the same way. The battle was joined again, and all the old arguments were reiterated.

Wilbur Mills was the primary force for Medicare in the House, and the Senate Finance Committee was the important decision-making body in the Senate. After Mills had introduced the concept that the costs of specialty services were to be divided, with the hospital cost under part A and the professional fee under part B, I was asked to go to Washington to explain to him the problems that hospitals would face under this arrangement. I spent half a day and received a very courteous reception. I tried to explain that, although arguments revolved around ethics and patient care, the issues seemed always to end up involving dollars. I expressed my concern that, if the hospital-based specialists were free to charge what the traffic would bear, the cost to patients and hospitals would skyrocket, and the ultimate consequence might well be total government control. To these I added my concern about the confusion this arrangement would cause for Medicare patients, the hospitals and the specialists themselves. I did not persuade Wilbur Mills. My concerns and cynicism were publicized in Richard Harris's 1966 book, *Medicare—A Sacred Trust*.[10]

The Senate Finance Committee was another matter. Senator Harry Byrd of Virginia was its chairman, and on the committee at that time were Paul Douglas, Abraham Ribicoff, Herman Talmadge, Everett Dirksen, Russell Long, and Maureen Neuberger of Oregon. I provided material to the committee through their staff leader, Jay Constantine, and was flattered that they used it as the basis for the Douglas Amendment and that

10. R. Harris, *A Sacred Trust*. New York: New American Library, 1966.

Senator Neuberger introduced my material into the Congressional Record. The Douglas Amendment would have placed all hospital-based specialties under part A and would have made their hospital reimbursement a component of the law. Paul Douglas and Abe Ribicoff wrote me that the arguments and the facts were compelling, and that not only they but the Senate Finance Committee and the Senate as a whole endorsed the Douglas Amendment. Unfortunately, when the Medicare bill came to a Senate-House conference, Wilbur Mills prevailed and the hospital-based specialty components wound up in part B.

This was considered a great victory by the hospital-based specialists. I was disappointed because I knew it would cause confusion in working relationships between hospitals and specialists and among patients covered by Medicare. I was also concerned about the potential cost increases. My fears were realized. Not only have health costs increased in certain areas more than anticipated, but confusion is rampant among the elderly patients and their families, as well as in hospital business offices and among physicians' secretaries. It is simpler for the physician: as a rule, he or she just submits the bill to the patient. By 1986, however, the state and federal governments were assuming far more authority in setting professional fees for Medicare patients, and this has not been received with enthusiasm by the medical profession.

However, patients' problems paying for hospital-based specialty services under the new Medicare legislation were immediate and nationwide. At Grace-New Haven, the specialty physicians on salary left it to the hospital business office and the intermediaries to deal with the coinsurance and the deductibles for part B. The patient still received a single bill for all hospital services. But things were different at hospitals where the physicians were not paid salaries or where they received a percentage of the gross departmental income. The division of part A and part B meant that elderly patients were confronted with two sets of bills, one from the hospital and one or many from the various professional specialties. Although 80 percent of the professional charges were covered by Medicare, the elderly patients were expected to pay 20 percent of these charges. To further complicate matters in a specialty such as clinical pathology, the professional involvement of the doctor was minimal. The doctor had nothing to do with examinations such as urinalyses or red blood counts. The hospital technician obtained the specimen, did the examination, and sent out the report, and the pathologist was only involved by virtue of having his or her name stamped on the report. I delighted in reminding the representatives of organized pathology that out of a $2.00 charge for a urinalysis, about $1.90 was the hospital cost. Ten cents might thus be considered the professional fee, which meant that they had the privilege of charging the patient 20 percent of this professional fee or two cents!

To hospital administrators' collective relief, this aspect of Medicare caused such universal confusion and dissatisfaction that, late in 1967, Congress amended the act to provide that radiologists and pathologists be paid 100 percent of their reasonable charges when these were included on the hospital bill. The professional components of radiological and pathological in-hospital services were thus to be reimbursed as if they were hospital services under part A, and not according to the co-payment provision of part B. The amendment brought Medicare in line with traditional practice. No other physician specialists were subject to this change.

Medicare has now been functioning for almost twenty years. Ironically, those who fought against a national health program for the aged have done quite well. So have the hospitals. The elderly, who were once clinic, ward, or service patients, unable to afford private care, have now shifted to private or semi-private pay categories. Unfortunately, as costs and charges rise, deductibles, co-insurance, and growing professional fees have become an increasing financial burden for the elderly patient. Legitimate concern is being voiced today about Medicare, its financial future, and its method of operation. I believe that it would have been expressed much earlier if not for the careful planning and development of health care plans for the elderly (particularly with regard to hospitalization) and the organization and administrative staffing that were developed to implement the legislation. It was not only the input of professionals like Arthur Hess and his associates but also the unique advisory board, the Health Insurance Benefits Advisory Council (HIBAC), that helped this program develop successfully. Careful preparation of the original legislation, retention of able staff, and a representative and experienced advisory board are three vital ingredients to the success of any government program.

I must admit to a certain prejudice in favor of the Medicare staff. My first introduction to them was at an early meeting in the fall of 1965 of representatives of the providers of Medicare services and the Medicare staff. This meeting turned out to be a most enjoyable affair, although it did not start that way. I represented the AHA and I was appalled to find that my organization had not done its homework and that I and an AHA staff assistant who also had not been briefed beforehand were expected to explain the program and needs of the AHA and its member hospitals with regard to the new legislation. The speaker of the AMA House of Delegates,

Milford O. Rouse, and members of the AMA board and staff, the presidents and executive officers of the organizations of pathologists, anesthesiologists, radiologists, physiatrists, medical schools, and every other conceivable provider was there—each with a prepared statement and specific recommendations.

Fortunately, I had sufficient background from my previous dealings with the AMA, the specialty boards, and the Douglas Amendment to discuss hospital needs and issues with relative authority. And there were not many immediate problems regarding part A of Medicare. However, I did not endear myself to some of my professional colleagues when I questioned the basis upon which some of the hospital-based specialists recommended their own reimbursements. The pathologists proposed a system in which each examination would be given a unit rating, depending on its complexity or difficulty. Medicare would be expected to reimburse the pathologists according to the established cash value per unit. The radiologists made essentially the same recommendation.

During the morning recess, I telephoned the hospital and asked that our laboratory and radiology activities for the previous year be analyzed according to their recommended unit ratings and charges. The results, which I reported to the group that afternoon, were rather startling. If the hospital had been reimbursed according to the pathologists' and radiologists' recommended formulae, it would have received many hundreds of thousands of dollars more than it did, although expenses would have been the same. I made myself even less popular when I pointed out that the professional component of the pathologists' fee for a blood count or a urinalysis amounted to ten cents. I did not know until almost twenty years later that Somers and Somers had quoted my calculations in their 1967 book.[11]

MEDICAID

Medicaid burst upon the hospital world as a bolt from the blue. The hospital component of Medicare had been discussed for years and various modifications had been explored before its enactment. But Title 19—the Medicaid Act—was a complete surprise to me and to most others in the health field. When it was being developed, I was asked by the AHA to meet with Ellen Winston, who was responsible for the administration of Medicaid, to try to convince her that separation of the hospital-based specialties and hospital charges was unwise. Dr. Crosby of the AHA told me

11. H. Somers and A. Somers, *Medicare and the Hospitals: Issues and Prospects*. Washington, D.C.: Brookings Institution, 1967, pp. 130–54.

that Medicaid could well have greater impact on the health and economic programs of this country than Medicare. I was no more successful with Dr. Winston than I had been with Wilbur Mills. Her predictable rejoinder to my arguments was that this had all been thrashed out in Medicare and she saw no reason to alter it now.

It is hard to reach any definitive conclusions about the relative impact of Medicare and Medicaid. Both have assumed great importance in the nation's health programs. But Medicaid legislation was developed with inadequate exploration of potential problems, the soundness or practicability of the program, its acceptibility to the providers, and particularly the willingness of the states to administer and finance the program. Unfortunately, states' ability to assume responsibility for Medicaid varied markedly, depending on their provision for administering health and welfare. I learned in Illinois that virtually all states had substantial deficiencies in this regard. Two decades after its legislation Medicaid still poses serious administrative and financial problems for government and the providers, as well as for those it is supposed to help. Yet it is still difficult today to envision clearly viable alternatives for a program that now involves so many persons who cannot afford to pay for their necessary health services.

It did not take long before my predictions of misunderstanding and confusion over Medicare were brought home to me directly, and I discovered that it was not just the elderly patient who had difficulty—it was the provider also. One day, a very intelligent and sincere woman of about eighty years of age came to my office with a whole sheaf of bills from our business office. She said that she did not understand them but wanted to pay what was proper. After looking them over, I said that I didn't understand them either. We made a date for a week later, at which time I promised to give her complete information. I then asked a senior resident, James Malloy, to work out the bills and educate me. It took him half a day to get all the facts, which he explained to me in great detail. It was all very complicated but I thought I understood it.

When the woman came back a week later, I told Mr. Malloy to listen while I tried to explain the bills to her. I did so with what I thought was clarity and precision. She nodded during my presentation and at the end asked me one question. I hadn't the slightest idea what the answer was, and I turned to Mr. Malloy and asked him to go on from there, which he did—for the next three-quarters of an hour. Finally, she told us that she hadn't the slightest idea what we were talking about and, though she was sure we knew what we were saying, she didn't think that she ever would. However, she was impressed with our sincerity and our obvious desire to be honest—so, if we would please tell her what she owed the hospital, she would make out a check.

I learned quickly from this experience and referred all subsequent questions on Medicare billing to my office staff. Not until my wife and I returned from Illinois and I started helping the widows of my friends with their Medicare forms did I realize that they, I, and even the secretaries in the doctors' offices were as confused as my elderly visitor of almost twenty years ago. As a rule, the hospital part is relatively simple (although objections and suspicions sometimes occur when the patient receives a long, detailed hospital bill stamped "THIS is not a BILL"). The problems that we have encountered have been with part B: the charge by the physician (including hospital-based specialists); the amount approved by Medicare, usually less than the physician's fee; the check from Medicare for 80 percent of the approved charge; and the second check for the other 20 percent, paid by the supplemental insurance that most elderly have. Some insurance carriers have a "piggy-back" arrangement with Medicare, so that Medicare automatically notifies the carrier of the supplemental insurance of Medicare's decision and the accepted professional fee. The supplemental carrier then sends a check for the additional 20 percent to the individual. But most insurance companies do not have this arrangement, and elderly patients and I have found it a most laborious process to get the proper information to the insurance company and then to identify the check when it arrives weeks later. The nurses in my personal physician's office have told me in despair that they used to spend 75 percent of their time working with patients as nurses. Now they are devoting 75 percent of their time helping their elderly patients with insurance forms.

I have come to know many of the Medicare staff in Connecticut by telephone, and I have found them uniformly courteous and helpful, but bound by rules and regulations coming from on high. Their difficulties are compounded by the fact that policies and regulations are being developed at higher and higher bureaucratic or administrative levels and further complicated by legislative interventions and constraints. Nor does the private sector help as much as it should. Instead, disagreement continues among those resources providing and financing health care. The added factor of competition is making solutions even more difficult. Home health care is an example of this which has particular pertinence to the aged.

HOME HEALTH CARE

My involvement with Medicare, the problems of the aged in Illinois, and the difficulties of the aged in dealing with Medicare were all preparations for my next phase of post-graduate education, which took place with the visiting nurse or home health care agency. I learned that this type of institution could be a vital component of a health system that was concerned with a continuum of care.

On our return from Illinois, my wife, who had previously been active on the board of the Hamden Public Health and Visiting Nurse Association, suggested that we both join the board of the Regional Visiting Nurse Agency (RVNA), which was an expansion of the Hamden agency that included the neighboring towns of North Haven, Woodbridge, and Bethany. I eventually became its president in 1978. As my wife and I became active on the board and I learned of the problems, finances, clientele, and services of this type of agency, I began to appreciate the significant role that it played in the health delivery system. It fit well into my evolving concept of a continuum of health care. First, however, I had to recognize that there were two broad types of home health agencies. Both were dependent upon the doctor for referral, orders, and follow-up, but otherwise they were different. One type was an extension of the doctor, existing solely to carry out his orders. If he ordered an injection or an enema, the nurse would go to the house and administer it. (I term these agencies "shot-nurse" or "enema-nurse" agencies.) The second type, which I was fortunate to find in the RVNA, also carried out specific orders, but went far beyond this to view the patient as a person in a home or a family, whose overall health was considered in relation to his or her social environmental context.

This important distinction was made clear to me when I spent a day accompanying one of the staff nurses on her rounds. I was profoundly impressed with the extent of her knowledge, not only of the patients' medical conditions, but also of their family situation, physical surroundings, the amount of help they needed for everyday living, and the range of social, economic, and environmental problems that affected their health needs. During this day, and from many subsequent conversations, I also became aware of many doctors' abysmal ignorance of the home conditions or other problems of the patient and the family. The practice of medicine has changed markedly during the last generation or two of physicians: time pressure and the requirements of diagnostic and therapeutic equipment have limited physicians' working environment more and more to their offices and institutions—particularly the hospital. Visiting patients' homes is now rare. When problems arise, it seems more efficient, convenient, and effective to have the patient come to the doctor's office or the emergency room.

Yet is is expensive and frequently inconvenient for the elderly patient to visit the doctor's office, and many problems cannot be solved over the phone. This is the situation in which a good visiting nurse or public health nurse is invaluable. Many problems that are not directly medical nevertheless affect the patient's overall welfare and can only be learned by direct contact. Experienced home health care nurses can provide the physician with their judgment of these problems and needs. They can also transmit the opinions or arrange for the services of other health care specialists. Physical, occupational, and speech therapists, dietitians, and social workers are all available through a well-organized and well-staffed home health care agency. Judgment of the type of skills required is also part of this service, so that home health aides can be used when appropriate, with supervision from visiting nurses as needed or indicated.

The professional home health supervisor is frequently in the best position to note a need and arrange for a service for a patient or family. Such services as homemakers, chore-persons, meals, transportation, and daycare may make it possible to continue to care for a patient at home—or even make such care unnecessary. This type of service outside the hospital building is an important and, until recently, often unrecognized or underutilized component in the delivery of health care. As I came to realize in Illinois, it is also one of the mechanisms by which health and social services can be efficiently brought into working relationship. Just as E. M. Bluestone used to refer to the hospital home care program as the "hospital without walls," I regard this function of such an agency as part of a more comprehensive "health care institution without walls."

This is no new discovery. Health care insurance agencies have for years been developing payment mechanisms for such services in lieu of or following hospitalization. This was done to encourage early hospital discharge and to diminish utilization of nursing homes. The increasing number of for-profit home care agencies is indicative of the demand. Yet the full potential of these agencies in caring for patients after hospital discharge is still not appreciated by the vast majority of physicians, whose professional orientation is still, with rare exceptions, directed toward acute care.

The most dramatic illustration of the value of the home health agency occurred by sheer coincidence at the annual meeting of the RVNA at which I was retired as president of the board. The program included a slide presentation by representatives of the various disciplines in the agency. They built their story around a specific patient, showing how the various personnel were involved. After the show they invited the patient to speak. I noticed that one of the nurses rather closely accompanied her to the podium, helped her up the stairs, and showed her how to adjust the microphone. I paid little attention since this seemed normal courtesy to a person unaccustomed to speaking in public. The attractive, middle-aged speaker succinctly and intelligently referred to the help she had received from the staff, and added that she did not know how she could have managed without their assistance. The presentation was obviously unrehearsed, but the sincerity and evident rapport between the woman and the nursing staff were gratifying. After the meeting, I congratulated her on her participation. She did not really look at me, however, and when she extended her hand to shake mine, it wasn't in quite the right direction. "I am sorry, Dr. Snoke," she said. "I can't see you—I am blind." I was taken by surprise. I subsequently learned that she had also lost both legs because of complications of diabetes, though I had not even suspected it as she went to the stage. She also had a mildly retarded daughter with cerebral palsy, and her husband had left her. She and her daughter lived alone, she ran her own household and was fiercely independent. It was clear that this would have been impossible without the help of the agency and her doctors—the latter involved primarily through the reports and visits of the RVNA staff and her visits to the clinic. This was an extremely impressive demonstration of the variety and quality of assistance that can be given by a people-oriented home health care service agency working with understanding physicians.

Although there is little argument today that home health care is a valuable and constructive component of the health service delivery system, it is remarkable how long the health system took in accepting this. Early in the deliberations about home care in 1948, E. M. Bluestone wrote about the extramural home-care function of the hospital. His words still ring true today, but it was not until 1980, over thirty years later, that the AHA Council on Patient Service reclassified a statement on the role and responsibilities of hospitals in home care as guidelines.

> The American Hospital Association and its member hospitals recognize home care as an element of continuing care, and as an essential component of comprehensive patient care. They accept their responsibility to foster the availability of home care services of high quality. No longer can a hospital's service program be defined in terms of in-patient care alone. The hospital must assume its proper responsibility to ensure a continuum of preventative, acute, rehabilitative, and long-term care wherever the patient may be. The extension of hospital service to the patient's home is both desirable and feasible when the patient's needs can be met there, and the home is suitable.[12]

I cannot criticize: it took me almost fifty years to recognize the potential

12. Council on Patient Service of the American Hospital Association, "Role and Responsibility of Hospitals in Home Care," *Guidelines*, 1980.

of the professional agency as an integral part of the continuum of health care.

The belated acceptance of the important role that home services should play in the health care system brings me back to Claudia Smith's 1983 thesis on services for the aged, which helped me to recognize the obvious. Society (both private and governmental) at the community, regional, state, and federal levels was now accepting the fact that the problems of the aged could no longer be ignored. As I read Miss Smith's description of the crazy quilt of services available to the elderly, I was impressed with the serious difficulties the elderly encountered in learning of the availability of such services—let alone locating or obtaining them. Eligibility requirements varied, and there were large gaps in mental health, adult daycare, and nutrition services. Transportation was a universal problem, and the services were forever changing. I used to admire those conscientious workers who carefully and meticulously prepared detailed guides of all the available resources for the aged with instructions on how to obtain help. But I also noted their frustration as they found that so many changes were taking place that the guide was out of date within a few months.

I started making my own list of services and facilities available to or required by the aged. I thought that I was relatively familiar with the "quilt" but, when I discussed my list with the director of the local agency for the aging and the senior staff of the RVNA, I realized how much I had to learn. They fleshed out my list substantially, and I have no doubt that theirs could be expanded as well.

1. Acute General Hospital Care
2. Long-Term Health Care
   a. Skilled nursing home care
   b. Long-term nursing home care
   c. Custodial nursing home care
3. Ambulatory Health care
   a. Doctors' offices
   b. Clinics
   c. Emergi-centers
   d. Surgi-centers
   e. Daycare for the frail
4. Home Health Care
   This is difficult to present in any uniform manner. The home health care agencies may be for-profit or nonprofit, and the services they provide may range from basic and traditional to broad and comprehensive.
   a. Visiting Nurse—Public Health and Nurse Practitioner
   b. Licensed Practical Nurse
   c. Home Health Aide

    d. Medical social service

    e. Occupational therapy

    f. Physical therapy

    g. Speech therapy

    h. Nutritionist or dietician

    i. Medical supplies and equipment

    j. Specialized therapy, such as intravenous therapy, specialized treatments, and so on

    k. Hearing aid

    l. Bereavement service

5. Home Care Services

    a. Chore person

    b. Homemaker

    c. Home help

    d. Friendly visiting

    e. Telephone reassurance

    f. Counselling

    g. Companion

    h. Bath aide

6. Nutrition

    a. Congregate meals

    b. Home delivered meals

    c. Shopping assistance

    d. Mobile markets

7. Housing

    a. From congregate housing, to assistance in individual or shared domicile.

8. Transportation for every conceivable purpose: shopping, professional visits, senior centers, adult daycare, recreation.

9. Respite Care

Short term care in the home to help those caring for the aged. This could be of all types—companion, housekeeper, health aide.

10. Legal Services

11. Mental Health Services

Ranging from home care to ambulatory care in offices and clinics to institutional care of all varieties.

12. Health Screening

    a. Audiology

    b. Vision

    c. Dental

    d. Diabetes, hypertension, and other specialized examinations

13. Energy

14. Protection

15. Hospice

This can be in an institutional facility for care of the dying. It can also be provided by the Hospice organization through a direct home health care service or in cooperation with a local home health care agency. Ironically, in some areas Hospice services are limited if the patient does not die when anticipated. The home health care agency may then return the patient to his or her home for continued agency care until death—or until the patient takes a turn for the worse.

This listing of the services and facilities needed by the aged is of value not only to document the magnitude and complexity of the system but also to point out two related questions.

How are the services financed?
How does the elderly patient or the family learn about and obtain these services?

Funding currently comes from government and private sources on every level—federal to local—and with an enormous variety of conditions. Although a number of sources fund specific, identified needs of the aged, variation in the type and quality of programs developed for the aged are frequently determined not necessarily by their specific needs but by the requirements of the potential source of funds. As Willie Sutton robbed banks because that was where the money was, local, regional, and even state programs cannot help but be influenced by the requirements or directions attached to the available funds. If the patient or some third party can be charged for some of the costs, so much the better. The problems of judiciously correlating legitimate needs of the aged with funds (which are clearly finite) has not yet been solved. I doubt whether it will be solved as long as there are so many agencies and jurisdictions, in the federal government, the states, and the municipalities, all vying for dollars and turf. The only polite comment I can make on the competency or quality of the services provided is that their variety appears to be almost infinite and identification and evaluation of these services limited.

Traditional nonprofit agencies, which used to provide most of the services to the elderly, are now finding commercial organizations entering this field in increasing numbers because government and insurance funds are more easily available. Hospitals, partly because of the DRG pressure for early discharge, and partly because a high percentage of their patients are elderly, are moving rapidly into the long-range health care system. As the hospitals place increased emphasis upon combined nonprofit and profit organizations, patients, their families, and their physicians must select from a confusing variety of options available for continuing care. The hospital is in the best position to coordinate and advise on services. However, as it develops its own profit divisions for pharmaceuticals, medical equipment and supplies, specialized treatments, and home health care programs, more commercial home health care programs are being developed and embraced by hospitals. What will be the relationship of these new programs with the traditional agencies?

Will they make available additional resources for organizing and providing needed health services, or will a two-tier system result?

It is, of course, possible for the knowledgeable aged person, family, or physician to arrange for needed services. But most families, and particularly elderly individuals or couples living alone, frequently know neither what they need nor how to find out. Sometimes they do not even realize they need help. Two types of organizations offer the possibility of a coordinated service approach. Cooperation between these agencies could be of great value to the hospital seeking to provide for a continuum of care, to the indigent or medically indigent, and to those who can pay. These organizations are the municipal elderly service agencies and the home health care agencies. With proper channels of communication, these two types of organization can be of great value in sorting out the complicated needs of the aged. The municipal elderly service departments have tremendous potential—if properly organized, staffed, and supported—not only in providing social services to the elderly and their families but also by stimulating formation of other services such as congregate housing, nutrition, transportation, information, counseling, recreation, and financial support to other direct social service agencies. Unfortunately, the caliber and competence of these local departments vary depending upon local elected officials as well as personnel. It seems surprising that federal and state agencies concerned with the aging do not put more pressure upon local communities to improve obviously inadequate staff and programs.

Voluntary nonprofit home health agencies have been the traditional and primary source of health services for the aged outside of institutions. The Connecticut RVNA, for example, is concerned with both health and social needs of the patient in his or her home. It is large enough to provide most services directly, and when necessary it arranges for additional services from other agencies—or if the proper encouragement and financing is available, it expands its own resources. It is particularly valuable as a professional liaison between the physician and the patient or family. This is particularly helpful in teaching them to cope with aging.

I am impressed with the potentially major role the home health care agencies can assume in caring for the aged in the home and keeping them out of institutions (acute or long-term) as long as possible. However, to carry out this role, these community home health agencies must

- concern themselves with the aged individual as a person, with social as well as health needs;
- be large enough to provide comprehensive service twenty-four hours a day;
- be able to refer the patient or family to the variety of other resources and services that the patient needs; and

• provide follow-up, maintain communication with the physician, and, when necessary, tactfully educate him or her.

(On the negative side, community home health agencies must also face discriminatory referral practices by hospitals, their main source of referrals. Hospitals may retain paying patients in their own profit-making systems.)

Connecticut developed a prototype of this kind of agency in a demonstration project started in 1974 as Triage.[13] It became the darling of the legislature and from it was developed a statewide case, assessment, and management (CAM) agency, Connecticut Community Care, Inc. (CCCI). Its objectives are essentially those that I have outlined, except that it does not provide patient services itself. Instead, it monitors the available programs, checks on the progress of those elderly individuals for whom it is able to accept responsibility, and, when possible, finances other program services from federal, state, or other funds. The organization has made a substantial contribution in emphasizing the value of a coordinating agency, when home health care agencies are not large or comprehensive enough to assume this responsibility themselves. But it may not be necessary or worth the cost of an additional layer in the health care system if the various state health and social service departments assist home health care agencies themselves to grow in size, competence, and vision. I hope that CCCI continues as a needle until all the home health care agencies become truly comprehensive. I am encouraged with the progress being made by the voluntary home health care agencies in expanding the scope and quality of their services.

The cost to the government of financing care for the aged and the cost of financing health care for employees are producing strange partnerships between government and industry. Both are becoming increasingly aware of the magnitude and the growing complexity, of all aspects of health care, and both are now looking carefully at the whole health care system. Unfortunately, their concern is primarily with costs— but perhaps this scrutiny will lead to improvement of the present system—or nonsystem.

This attention may eventually be beneficial to all—and particularly the elderly—if only the dollar sign does not obliterate the human needs of the patient. The aged are an ideal group to demonstrate the interrelationship of the social and health problems, which, to be solved, require a far more organized and coordinated program than has yet appeared.

13. M. Shealy, "Triage—Coordinated Delivery of Services to the Elderly," Executive Summary, December, 1979. Joan Quinn and J. Segal, *Coordinated Community Services for the Elderly* (New York: Springer, 1982).

However, I question whether any simplistic solution such as competition will provide a system which will allow the appropriate agency or agencies to survive and provide the best care to people. Competition and profit-making are too easily confused, and the former too easily leads to the destruction of community-oriented agencies or the creation of a two-tier health care system. The obvious example is the "dumping syndrome" found in many large communities, but it can be much more subtle. I have already commented on the hospital-based approach which unabashedly creates a proprietary home health care agency with profit-making subsidiaries such as pharmacies, medical supplies, and intravenous solutions in the home—all as partners with the hospital and geared to the private pay and third-party reimbursement system. The one government agency that should be supporting community-based home health care agencies is the Health Care Financing Administration of HHS, but this agency is not doing its job. The HCFA has embraced the DRG pricing approach, which stimulates early discharge of Medicare patients from the acute care hospital. Under this approach greater involvement of the home health care agency appears logical and necessary. However, local home health care agencies are encountering increased difficulty both in obtaining approval for the care of these patients and in getting prompt reimbursement. At first I thought this might be a problem of a few specific agencies, until I talked with the intermediaries and found that it appeared to be the attitude of the national HCFA.

One wonders if HCFA is ignoring the overall care of the aged Medicare patients, looking instead at the cost of each component without reference to the entire cost of care. The agency has expressed criticism and alarm over the recent increase in the use of home health care agencies and the resultant expense to Medicare for their services. But what else is expected from pressure on hospitals to discharge patients earlier? Elderly patients on Medicare (as well as many younger patients) need some type of follow-up care. They do not become automatically self-sufficient after being wheeled out of the hospital.

Local home health care agencies are having to provide more sophisticated care more frequently because patients are sicker when they are discharged from the hospital. But agency expenses are increased not only because of the type of services they are delivering to these patients but also because more reporting and justification of these services is required. The agencies are becoming more liable to criticism and delayed or refused payment by the intermediaries, as a result of the more extensive questioning stimulated by the HCFA bureaucracy. To make matters worse, these more complicated reports are required to be submitted in a "timely" and correct fashion. If this is not done to the satisfaction of the HCFA and its intermediaries, the helpful system of periodic interim payments may be withdrawn if mistakes exceed a certain percentage. This does not seem unreasonable—except that refusals of payment are often found to be due to the intermediary's errors, not the home agency's. Medicare patients make up a substantial proportion of the case load of many voluntary, community health care agencies. Delays in payments impair their cash flow, which can be devastating.

One cannot help suspecting that these complicated HCFA requirements are a bureaucratic technique to avoid or delay payments. As a final result, patients may be forced into health care facilities for which Medicare is not responsible, such as long-term nursing homes. The AHA *Hospital Week* of April 26, 1986, reported that at a recent meeting of the House Ways and Means Committee's health subcommittee, HCFA Acting Associate Administrator Kevin Moley said contractor claims payment periods were to be increased. The lead article of the AMA *News* of May 2, 1986, carried the headline "HCFA Sanctions Medicare Claims Slowdown." It stated the current policy very simply:

> Despite earlier assurances that the current 1986 Medicare claims processing budget would not require slowdowns in payments to physicians, hospitals, and patients, Medicare officials now admit that a claim slowdown is inevitable. Furthermore, the Reagan Administration has decided that such holdups are a desirable way of doing business, and will tell the companies that process Medicare claims to continue the lags again next year, even if more money becomes available. The aim is to use the "float" to increase the amount of interest the government earns on Medicare trust funds by about $130 million a year.

I did not want to believe this and asked for confirmation from the House Ways and Means Health Subcommittee. I regret to say that the report was confirmed. I am sorry, for this seems an unfair way for bureaucracy to approach the complicated system of caring for people for whom society has accepted an obligation.

Some home health care agencies are undoubtedly inadequate in services or reporting, and of course HCFA and the intermediaries should expect accuracy and efficiency from providers. But the providers, in turn, should expect the same. Accordingly, I confess I enjoy the discomfort of some intermediaries when I question them about the delays in approval and payments and ask them whether HCFA's rule that the intermediary received one dollar for every five saved in provider payments is an example of good professional judgment, improved administration—or bribery!

I am also concerned that the Connecticut General Life Insurance

Company has decided to withdraw after twenty years from being the Part B Medicare intermediary for Connecticut. It is probable that Connecticut Blue Cross and Blue Shield, which has served as the Part A intermediary during this same period, will not want to assume this responsibility. The same pattern is developing in HCFA of having only one intermediary for home health care agencies in each of the ten HHS regions. If a single regional agency can function efficiently and effectively, this is fine. However, it is difficult to understand the pressure from Washington to locate the intermediary agency for New England in Maine. This agency now deals with fewer than ten home health care agencies. But Connecticut and Massachusetts both have more than one hundred—and there are approximately seventy more in Vermont, New Hampshire, and Rhode Island. In addition, the home health care agencies in New England have been told to prepare for the use of a computer system to deal with the intermediaries, and the Maine agency is inexperienced in this area. With all respect to the potential effectiveness of my Maine neighbors, I foresee cash flow and approval problems resulting from this type of centralization. The agencies' survival may be threatened with the increased load of referrals in combination with the ability of the Maine intermediary to process this added load.

As I questioned the local RVNA and the Connecticut Medicare intermediary for home health care about the increasing antipathy of HCFA, I heard of the report prepared by the National Association for Home Care on "The Attempting Dismantling of the Medicare Home Health Benefit." The report reflects very closely the phenomena that I have been observing in local home health care agencies during the past few months. It also contrasts the billions of dollars saved on hospital expenditures with the relatively modest increases in the costs for home health care, and it details the apparent influence of OMB upon the attitude of HHS and HCFA. I feel as if I have been transported back to 1975, when Charles Edwards resigned as the HEW assistant secretary for health and expressed his frustration with the health professionals dealing with OMB.[14] Whether this report of the National Association for Home Care to Congress and the appointments in 1986 of Dr. Bowen as secretary of HHS and William Roper as the head of HCFA will bring a more realistic and understanding approach to the system of caring for individuals after they have been discharged quicker and sicker from the hospitals remains to be seen. I hope that it will, for the care of the aged may well be an extremely important factor in encouraging this nation's attention on our overall health care system—or

14. C. E. Edwards, Memorandum to HEW Secretary Caspar Weinberger, December 1974, quoted in *The New York Times*, February 3, 1975.

nonsystem. If it can stimulate improved organization, administration, and leadership in the government and contribute to the development of a more effective, efficient and economical program for care, this will be a great contribution. If those responsible for the delivery of service also recognize the necessity of effective organization for a continuum of care, this will also be an important contribution for all the people in this nation.

12

Ethics

This is a difficult chapter to write, for I must discuss these subjects from a personal point of view, formed in large part from my own experiences, and many of my attitudes may be out of date. Although many of my decisions in the past were determined by the circumstances at that particular point in my education or career, underlying most of my actions was a growing concern for the care of people.

RIGHT TO HEALTH

During the debates on Medicare, as we worked with the Health Insurance Benefits Advisory Committee (HIBAC), Arthur Hess and his associates on the government Medicare staff, and the many providers (mostly voluntary) to establish regulations and procedures for the care of the aged, a storm arose when Milford O. Rouse, president of the AMA in 1967–68, was quoted as stating that health care was a privilege, not a right. I believe that Dr. Rouse was unfairly saddled with what was perceived as a heartless philosophy, for I later carefully read and reread the speech in which he supposedly made the statement, and it was not so dogmatic as first interpreted. However, the issue of privilege versus right was very much in the air at the time. My answer was simple. Health care was a right—the only problem was how to accomplish it. From the time of my medical education through my years in hospital administration, there had never been any doubt that all patients should receive adequate care. All patients received the same type of nursing, food, visiting hours, drugs, and special services. Those who wanted to pay for amenities such as single rooms, special nurses, and personal physicians, obtained them. But I never felt that ward patients in the hospitals with which I was associated—

in which the many interns and residents were supervised by faculty or attending physicians—received inferior care.

I never worried whether there was a constitutional or legal right to health care. My philosophy, and that of my associates was that there was an ethical and social right to adequate health care. The question then came down to the definition of what made up adequate health care. Unfortunately, this has become a serious dilemma because of ever-increasing costs and limited resources. Although these are serious problems today, they are not new. I had to face them almost forty years ago.

PENICILLIN

The worst period in my career was in 1946 and 1947. The war was over, personnel were more available, and penicillin (which had been first administered to a civilian patient in the United States in the New Haven Hospital in 1942) was now available in limited quantities and at high cost. It was clearly life-saving in certain cases, and its appropriateness for a number of other illnesses was being considered. Over 50 percent of Grace-New Haven's patients were either on welfare or in a ward category, and the full costs of their treatment were not paid. The hospital was running a large deficit, and we now had available a life-saving drug at the cost of $200 to $500 a day. (At that time, the average daily cost of the hospital room was around $10.)

Because of our financial situation, any major expenditure for penicillin had to be approved by the administration if the family could not guarantee payment. Thus I had the responsibility of meeting with the attending resident, chief of service, and whomever else seemed appropriate, and asking several simple questions. What is the diagnosis? How much penicillin a day should be given? What will be the cost to the hospital per day? For how many days will the therapeutic dosage be necessary? What are the chances that the drug will cure the patient? I then had to decide whether to allow the doctors to proceed with penicillin treatment. Frequently, the patient was a child or a young adult, which made my dilemma worse. It took many months for the cost of the drug to come down and for the doctors to become more familiar with the indications and the possible results. In the meantime, I had no one else to whom to pass the buck. I felt as if I were playing God, and, while I bent over backwards to approve the expenditures, those who died without the medication, as well as those who died after having received it, continued to haunt me.

Although I enlisted my colleagues as much as possible in my penicillin decisions, I was never able to organize a formal review group, which apparently took place in Seattle when renal dialysis first became available and the demand exceeded the available resources. They set up a screening committee of lay and professional persons, which was probably as fair and logical a method of deciding who should live and who should die as one involving laws, lawyers, judges, and courts. But my penicillin decisions were, at the beginning, based upon the best advice I could get from those I trusted professionally, as well as consideration of the slim financial resources of the hospital.

CONTRACEPTION AND ABORTION

Contraceptives and abortions did not affect my professional consciousness until I came to Connecticut. There was a strong Catholic influence in Massachusetts and Connecticut, which were the last remaining states to prohibit the prescription of contraceptives. Abortion was also frowned upon unless it could be demonstrated that it was necessary to preserve the life of the mother or the unborn child. (No one was ever able to explain to me the sense of a clause that permitted aborting a fetus to save its life.) Contraceptives were prescribed in our OB-GYN clinic, by private physicians, and in Planned Parenthood clinics throughout the state, but there was always the potential of legal action because of the outdated law. I followed with great interest the original effort to obtain a judgment on the Connecticut contraceptives law, which went to the Supreme Court only to be dismissed because of a lack of actual enforcement. So Estelle Griswold, executive director of the Connecticut Planned Parenthood League, and Lee Buxton, chairman of the Department of Obstetrics and Gynecology of the Yale School of Medicine, undertook to prescribe contraceptives in their Planned Parenthood clinic and to publicize this widely so as to force the Connecticut authorities to take legal action and thus meet the Supreme Court's requirement. I invited Dr. Buxton and Mrs. Griswold to my office to discuss the possibility of the hospital clinic formally and publicly doing what we had been doing routinely but quietly. Their attorneys from the Yale Law School, Thomas Emerson and Catherine Roraback, concurred, and I discussed the plan individually with members of the hospital board. All seemed to agree, but when I brought up the plan at the next board meeting, someone worried that the hospital or university might lose its tax exemption. The argument was vague, but to my disgust, the board solemnly voted to abstain. Mrs. Griswold and Dr. Buxton went ahead and were arrested, giving the Supreme Court grounds to consider the case. Eventually, the Court declared the Connecticut laws on contraception unconstitutional.

Abortions were a much more difficult matter for the hospital and the physician. Obviously, no problem was presented in the care of spontaneous abortions or miscarriages, but a voluntary abortion was quite a different matter. Although the state law permitted abortions when necessary to save the life of the mother, no hospital had any formal procedure (at least that it would admit to) by which such an operation could be considered and approved. I always tried to support any woman who believed that the life of the fetus should be preserved, but I never could personally accept the philosophy that the life of the fetus took precedence over the life of the mother. This was even more disturbing to me when the woman already had one or more children. But I believed that the decision should be made by the pregnant woman herself. Of course, in those days one could not be associated very long with hospitals without becoming familiar with the case of the pregnant woman who had gone to an abortionist and then had to be brought to the emergency department because of life-threatening hemorrhage or infection.

In the late 1940s through the 1960s, "abortion on demand" was not an issue of which I was conscious, but abortions for medical reasons seemed appropriate, and it seemed proper for the hospital to make such operations available. Our procedure was quite straightforward and open. The patient's personal physician and the obstetrician would, at the patient's request, formally request a therapeutic abortion on her behalf. They would present the case to a committee of five—the chiefs of the university and the community obstetric and gynecology services, two specialists in the field covering the medical condition that seemed to warrant abortion, and me as the hospital administrator. The patient's physician would present the case, satisfy the committee of the patient's desire to undergo an abortion after counseling, and answer whatever questions were posed by the group. Sometimes decisions were deferred pending further investigation. Patients with malignancies, severe heart disease, and kidney disease were readily approved, although I can recall at least one case with hematuria and proteinuria in which permission was refused because we suspected that the patient had orthostatic albuminuria and vestiges of menstrual bleeding. She eventually delivered a normal baby.

The most difficult cases were those with psychiatric diagnoses, in which the entire family situation and future state of the child, the mother, and the family had to be taken into account. Adoption was considered and urged if the medical condition was not considered life-threatening. We had, of course, no authority if the patient decided to go elsewhere. Studies revealed that approximately 50 percent of the abortions were for psychiatric reasons, and my recollection is our reviews of the cases were professionally defensible, with perhaps the one following exception.

During the early years that we were doing this type of abortion, it was carried out openly at Grace-New Haven, but only rarely in most other Connecticut hospitals. I became aware of this when I learned at a cocktail party of a nurse who had been raped while visiting a patient and was pregnant. I asked if she was planning to have an abortion and was rather surprised to learn that none of the hospitals from Norwalk down to the New York line would perform one. But the woman wanted an abortion and was apparently searching for an abortionist. At the same party were a psychiatrist friend and the associate professor of obstetrics. They thought we should follow through, so I called the director of the hospital involved and asked him to get in touch with the woman and her doctor, who, if they wished, could refer her to my associates. The young woman and her doctor called me that afternoon. She was admitted to the psychiatric division, the committee met the next day, and after the story was told one question was asked. "Was there a possibility that this woman might commit suicide, if the baby were brought to term?" The answer was yes. Approval for the abortion was unanimous, and it was performed. There may be some who would disagree with our decision, but we considered our actions appropriate at that time, and I still do. I think that, from the time the hospital started making abortions possible, I and the leaders of the medical staff were slowly developing the philosophy that a woman should have the right to terminate her pregnancy if it could be shown that such an action was in her best interest. The committee did refuse some abortions because we felt there was no medical reason—organic or psychiatric. Some of these women went out of state or to an abortionist. Others, after counseling, went on to have their babies.

I am very disturbed by the militancy of some foes of abortion and birth control today. The American Life Lobby, for example, is, according to its brochure, "opposed to any birth control . . . being provided to the unmarried—be they adolescent or otherwise." In addition, their president states that "life begins at the moment of fertilization . . . and abortion should never be a solution to any problem"—including the problem of a pregnant twelve-year-old, or that of a woman who has been raped. These rigid attitudes seem to me to show no respect for the quality of life, or for the decisions that people and their doctors must make considering all the factors of the individual situation.

STERILIZATION

Sterilization never seemed to be of much concern—either publicly or professionally—when compared to contraceptives or abortions. It was not until I came to Connecticut that I recall the medical board or the hospital administration taking any official action in these matters. If a man wished a vasectomy, his surgeon would usually perform it. We heard occasionally of a man who wanted a vasectomy undone—then the discussion was usually about the chances of successful reversal. Sterilization of women was another story. I never could quite understand why tubal ligations were more carefully considered and more frequently refused than vasectomies—but our attitudes toward the two sexes were substantially different. Many physicians hesitated to do any tubal ligations during a woman's child-bearing years.

I thought it would be wise to set up some sort of guidelines to be of assistance in counseling patients who desired sterilization. (This was much more important before the birth control pill became widely used.) A representative group of various specialties on the medical staff, social service workers, and the hospital board developed the guidelines. They were broad and emphasized individual decision, counseling, the age of the woman, and the number of children already in the family. For example, a woman of twenty-five years of age and one child would not be considered appropriate for tubal ligation without other unusual medical conditions. However, sterilization of a woman of thirty-five years of age with five or more children was usually approved.

I was not completely aware of the value of this unofficial policy until a close friend cornered me at a Christmas party and started giving me hell for the stuffy, restrictive rules of the hospital regarding sterilization. We went off in a corner, and he told me that his wife was pregnant with their sixth or seventh child. They had asked her obstetrician to ligate her tubes after this pregnancy but he had refused, stating that the hospital rules would not permit it. I knew of their large family, for my wife and her friend had discussed their apparent inability to prevent pregnancy. I met with her obstetrician the next day and reminded him that he was a member of the group that had established the flexible ground rules, and that the woman met the criteria for approval of sterilization. I asked if he or I should so inform the couple. There was no debate. He said that he would talk with them and do the procedure after the pregnancy.

RELIGION

When I became Assistant Director of Strong Memorial Hospital, I was profoundly impressed with Gregory Dugan, a Catholic priest who considered the hospital and its patients to be his parish. He was there night and day visiting all the patients listed as Catholic on the hospital admitting forms, and he came to my office whenever he had problems. We became close friends because of his obvious concern for the welfare of all the patients, and because we both respected the beliefs of the other. Father Dugan's unique contribution was his interest in all the patients in the hospital. My wife, following the birth of each of our sons, was particularly impressed with his encouraging visits to the young mothers. His interest in people, as well as his understanding of the hospital's needs, were particularly valuable when the resident staff needed help to get an important autopsy permission. If the family were Catholic and hesitant, I would explain the situation to Father Dugan. When he and I were in agreement, he would go with me to talk with the family. Usually, we got the permission.

In New Haven, I had the administrative responsibility to see that all faiths were properly supported. I found a complicated situation. Directly across from the hospital was St. John's, with an impressive number of young, eager, active Catholic priests. As was the custom in most hospitals, our admitting office routinely inquired the religion of the patient, which was noted on his or her chart. Every Catholic patient was visited and his or her progress followed by these young men. Protestants had the same attention if they were from the area and members of a particular church. But many patients came from out-of-town, and many said they were Protestants but did not go to any particular church. These patients were considered the responsibility of the Protestant chaplain assigned to this jurisdiction by the local Protestant Council of Churches. The Protestant chaplains were almost always pleasant, elderly, semi-retired ministers. For over ten years, with one exception, Protestant patients were served by these elderly, well-meaning, but rather ineffective clerics.

I had trouble with one long-time hospital custom. Whenever a Catholic patient was placed upon the danger list, the Catholic priest would automatically be notified. When this happened, he would consider the patient in danger of dying and would appear to provide Extreme Unction. This custom put me in the middle of a battlefield. Several times a year, I would be called to referee a confrontation between a young Catholic priest and a member of the resident staff. The priest believed it was his duty to give the last rites to the patient, but the doctor occasionally felt that, if the patient believed he or she were in danger of dying, it would adversely affect his or her attitude or prognosis. Sometimes emotions ran so high that the discussion almost came to blows. Each case required a different type of adjustment, and I enjoyed none of them. (The Catholic priests later solved the problem by changing the connotation of Extreme Unction to "anointing the sick.")

The problems continued until I was fortunate enough to have both the dean of the Yale Divinity School and a hospital board member who was president of the City Missionary Society in New Haven in the hospital as patients at the same time. They were both disturbed by the Protestant minister, and I took the advantage to propose that, if the Divinity School would provide an academic appointment and the Missionary Society would underwrite the salary, the hospital would provide a secretary and office for a hospital chaplain. There was quick agreement, a search committee was established, and Edward Dobihal was appointed Protestant chaplain for the hospital. My dividends from the appointment were numerous, and some unexpected. First, I could resign from the unwanted task of reconciling the resident staff and the priests on the subject of Extreme Unction. Rev. Dr. Dobihal adjusted the definitions of what was required for a patient on the danger list, and interpreted to non-Catholic members of the house staff the feelings of the priests. He took over as the full-time Protestant chaplain and quickly developed a close, friendly, working relationship with the Catholic priests across the street, the other Protestant ministers in the area, and the rabbis. Another extra dividend was his development of a hospital chaplaincy program that attracted Protestants, Catholic priests and nuns, and rabbis. In addition, Rev. Dr. Dobihal and his wife, Shirley, brought an interest in the new philosophy of hospice. The Yale School of Nursing had invited Dame Cicely Saunders to the nursing school for four weekly seminars on the hospice programs she had developed at St. Christopher's Hospital in London. The experience was remarkable. Dr. Saunders moved from a small classroom in the school of nursing to the largest auditorium in the medical school, all due to the remarkable interests of the medical center in her program.

The Dobihals took a six months' sabbatical to visit St. Christopher's in 1970–71 and then returned to help stimulate one of the first hospice programs in this country. By this time, I was working with the governor of Illinois. I arranged in 1972 to have the Dobihals come to the University of Illinois Medical Center in Chicago for a day's conference on hospice. The intense interest of the nurses, social workers, interns, residents, and faculty of the medical center impressed me even as I recalled the earlier interest shown in Dr. Saunder's visit to New Haven.

RIGHT TO DIE

The whole subject of the right to life and the right to die has become far more complicated in the 1980s than it was in the 1930s and 1940s, partly due to the aging of the population and the professional advances in saving and prolonging life. I suspect that there is also a substantial increase in the numbers and in the noise level of those who not only have strong feelings about their own welfare and future but also believe that their personal opinions must be shared by others. My philosophy has not changed over my professional career. However, my attitude today, which might be described by a charitable individual as liberal or permissive, is unfortunately complicated by militant "pro-life" individuals, and by courts, judges, laws, and fears of legal or financial penalties. Perhaps they are correct—I don't agree.

When I was a resident at Stanford, one of my patients was an older woman with recurrent metastases from cancer. She was in agony every time she drew a breath. I knew what I believed should be done, and discussed it with the woman, her husband, and my chief of service. We found ourselves in complete agreement. I ordered sufficient morphine to keep the patient comfortable and drowsy, and stopped everything else. She died in comfort. I have always believed that I did the best for her, but there is no question that I shortened her life. Recently I told this story to a physician in active practice, whom I admire for his respect for the welfare of his patients. He understood and concurred with what I had done, but he said that today such an action would put me in jeopardy. This was long before the living will, which has been highly publicized in recent years. There are still those who oppose its purpose and its philosophy. I support their right to their philosophies, but disagree with their seeking to impose their beliefs upon others. Death with dignity and comfort should be the prerogative of any person who desires it. Prolongation of life in acute discomfort—particularly through the employment of heroic and expensive measures that cannot reverse the inevitable end—should require extraordinary justification.

Three of the men I admired most and who had helped me generously when I came to New Haven, developed serious arteriosclerosis in their later years. Disoriented, blind, completely helpless, and unaware of their families or friends, all these men existed for a number of years. I visited them occasionally and sat, watched, and suffered, thinking of their independence, their concern for the welfare of others, and their many contributions to the community and to me over the years. I could not believe that they would have wanted this type of existence, which custom, philosophy, or their families prescribed for them.

I became the legal conservator of a close relative of my wife whom I had known and respected for her help and affection for my wife and her contributions to programs for the blind. She developed Alzheimer's disease and drifted further and further from reality. Eventually, she recognized no one and refused to eat. My wife and I visited her regularly in the nursing home and knew that she was being cared for conscientiously and with kindness. I told the staff and her attending physician that extraordinary or heroic procedures were not to be instituted without notifying me. The implications were clear—and, to make sure, I specifically talked about not using antibiotics for such complications as pneumonia. Years later, metastases of a previous breast cancer appeared. No new therapy was initiated, and she quietly died a few months later. I believed that I had repaid her for at least some of her contributions to my wife and to the blind, and I also felt that she would have approved of what I had not done.

There are so many variations of hopeless or terminal illness. Some are in constant pain; and others seem to be in a continued state of apprehension and fear. The courts may well take more responsibility for setting criteria and deciding whether to allow people to die. Legal guidelines are valuable, but a representative group of compassionate people from medicine, religion, and social sciences, after consultation with the family and particularly, if possible, the patient, is more likely to arrive at an equitable, compassionate, and humane decision. Physicians, as a rule, agree that it is valuable to include other disciplines in this decision-making process. I am always impressed with the determination of physicians to save or preserve life. But when the situation appears hopeless, outside support and confirmation is welcome.

Two occurrences over the past few years have helped me clarify my viewpoint on the problems of prolongation of life and the issues of ethics, law, and economics. Each has, in its own way, illustrated the issue as one of considering the patient as a unique person in an environment with infinite demands and finite resources and a part of a family that also deserves consideration. The case of Karen Anne Quinlan is well known. I have nothing but respect for the parents of this young woman in their steadfast support for her welfare and their realistic appraisal of the hopelessness of her recovery. Their courage and that of the court, in the face of widespread publicity, in approving the removal of the life support system with the expectation that she would die, is remarkable. That Miss Quinlan did not die and remained in a coma for years until her death in 1985 was not expected, but was accepted and supported. I do not believe that anything should be done to change such a situation other than not ordering additional heroic measures to preserve life. The financial implications of Miss Quinlan's care were real, but the feelings of her family took precedence.

As those who support life and oppose contraception and abortion under any circumstances continue to press their views and requirements upon others, I believe they are in danger of forgetting the quality of life into which a child may be born as well as the effect upon the remainder of the family. It was relatively easy to assist a girl of eleven or twelve years old to deliver a baby that she understood to be a doll, but it was the girl's mother who had the responsibility of taking care of both children, as well as the rest of her family. I do not believe anyone should have the right to force this situation upon others who do not share their convictions.

The parents' agony during the prolonged efforts to preserve the life of a premature baby is remarkably related in Robert and Peggy Stinson's book, *The Long Dying of Baby Andrew*.[1] The baby was born in 1976. He weighed one pound, twelve ounces, and was almost sixteen weeks premature. A conflict arose between the parents and the hospital, whose doctors assumed responsibility for prolonging—at a terrible price—the life of an infant that virtually no one had good reason to think would survive and grow up normally. I can well understand the professional challenges this tiny baby presented to the medical and nursing staff—this was why I supported the acute care neonatal unit at Grace-New Haven. But it was a mistake to regard parents as extraneous factors, unimportant compared to the challenge of the battle for the life of Baby Andrew. I only hope that those who cared for Baby Andrew now understand better the parents' long, emotionally draining experience, and that the couple tried for another child.

A happier experience occurred in the University of Chicago Medical Center. A mother of three was transferred to the Lying-In Hospital Unit with a diagnosis of diabetes, twins at seven months, which were estimated to weigh about a pound and a half each, and signs of premature labor. The problem was how to give her medication to prevent the premature delivery and still keep her feeling well and interested in life. In this case, the institution was flexible enough to adapt its policies to adjust to the needs of the family. They provided a homelike, supportive atmosphere in which the family and the hospital staff could care for the woman—knowing that each week delivery could be delayed the twins would be enabled to grow and develop. The result was the delivery of two babies, five pounds, thirteen ounces and six pounds, five ounces, some two months later—just one week early. It is a heartwarming story, deservedly well-publicized in Chicago and with the kind of happy ending that hospitals, doctors, and nurses delight in.

It is obviously difficult for the hospital and the staff to adjust to the

1. Robert and Peggy Stinson, *The Long Dying of Baby Andrew*. (New York: Little Brown, 1979.)

myriad of different situations and do the best for all individuals concerned. The examples of Baby Andrew and the Peres twins reflect the problems faced by society and by the medical professions as more emphasis is being placed upon handicapped infants and a variety of governmental regulations appear to be on their way. We must ask ourselves whether advances in medical science have outstripped our social objectives related to the quality of patient care. Perhaps now there should be a second small statuette, called "Discharged Living," to remind us again that we are responsible not only to the patient, but to the family for the results of our care.

I have always been ready to use all available resources to preserve the life of the young. (My mother was born a two- or three-pound premature in 1875, and her Danish parents used the oven as her incubator!) My pediatric experience was continually a stimulus to help the young live and develop, and this background encouraged my conviction of the value of the acute care neonatal unit in Grace-New Haven. Its staff has become able to care for ever smaller and younger infants. However, this may be a double-edged sword, in that some babies may have survived to live lives of poor quality—babies who, years ago, would have died because sophisticated care was not available. Those insisting upon extreme efforts to save newborns must recognize the potential financial and emotional problems for the patient and the family. As we pass rules, regulations, and laws, and make professional decisions, we must recognize that our actions do not take place in a vacuum—we must consider the continuum of life and care as well as the limit to our resources.

13

Conclusion:
Establishing a National Health Policy

The past fifty years have brought striking developments in our therapeutic armamentarium and in our approaches to the care of people. Until recently changes came about gradually, but, in the last decade or so, the transformation has occurred with almost explosive speed. Techniques, administration, organization, and, most particularly, costs are changing at an exponential rate. I have found it difficult, on the one hand, to imagine the potential effect of these changes on health care and, on the other hand, to avoid pontificating in these pages upon their implications. I cannot resist observing, however, that our chief preoccupation today appears to be with costs, controls, marketing, competition, profit-making, and cost effectiveness—in short, with the "bottom line." This fundamental shift in philosophy seems to bode ill for the concept that patients are people and that we, as well as they, will be poorer if we forget it.

I think we all know that something needs to be done. But what is that something? Over many years I have often criticized my colleagues in the health establishment—of which I have been a part—over inadequacies of the current system. I have described its components as fragmented, inexplicably related, improperly planned, and poorly administered. Occasionally I have suggested partial remedies or pointed to certain accomplishments. But I have never been able to propose a comprehensive solution to the problems I have raised. (Neither, in my judgment, has anyone else.) I have not proposed such a solution here. I have only illustrated, mainly from my own experience in the field, how desperately it has been—and still is—needed.

If solutions are to be found, they will come only from the efforts of dedicated and imaginative representatives of every aspect of health care working together with open minds and unswerving determination. That has yet to happen. Not long ago the Commonwealth Fund gave a small planning grant to Yale's Department of Epidemiology and Public Health to set up a conference. Its objective was summarized as "the presentation of the necessary, interrelated, administrative components of a comprehensive, national health insurance program that should be taken into consideration as the decision-makers consider the various options. This is necessary so that there will be reasonable assurance that the programs or the steps of the program finally developed will have the optimum opportunity for flexibility and for success." The conference was not successful, for most of the discussions were dominated by advocates of specific programs who enjoyed debating their respective merits rather than examining basic administrative and organizational strategies with an eye to implementing a national health policy.

Nevertheless, I still believe that any approach to a nationwide health program must be massive, multidisciplinary, and integrated if it is to succeed. We might begin by developing a comprehensive list of questions on basic issues—social, economic, and political, as well as medical—the answers to which might suggest a way to establish a national health policy. We could then begin to implement solutions.

- What will this nation's health policy be? Should policy be determined by the states, or should there be basic national principles regulating the states' health legislation?
- Is health a right or a privilege?
- Should we separate health from social services?
- Are expenses for care increased by duplication, fragmentation, and unwieldy bureaucracy?
- Where can we find answers to these questions?
- How can we obtain and *retain* competent professionals to carry out health and social service programs?
- There are many people in this nation whose expertise, insight, and imagination could make invaluable contributions to this kind of exploratory examination. Supporting such a venture would be a fit project for one of our great foundations. A preliminary conference could prepare the way for appointment of a national commission on health policy comparable in scope and nonpartisan independence to the Hoover Commissions of 1953 and 1955.[1] Such a commission would have to be free to investigate the problems of health care and inseparably related issues without the handicap of having to represent special interests.

1. The Hoover Commission on Organization of the Executive Branch of the Government, established by Public Law 108, 83d Congress, July 10, 1953; and the second Hoover Commission, whose Task Force on Federal Medical Service reported in 1955.

From this body we could expect firm recommendations for a program that would integrate the efforts of many sectors, public and private, that are, or should be, concerned with the health and welfare of the population. The impressive Health Policy Agenda developed by the AMA may make a major contribution to such a goal. I believe, however, that finding the most widely acceptable solutions will require the work of a broader group.

Index